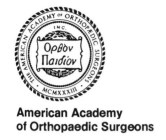

**American Academy
of Orthopaedic Surgeons**

Orthopaedic Science

A Resource and Self-Study Guide for the Practitioner

SYLLABUS

The material presented in this *Orthopaedic Science Syllabus* has been made available by the American Academy of Orthopaedic Surgeons for educational purposes only. This material is not intended to represent the only, or necessarily best, methods or procedures for the medical situations discussed, but rather is intended to present an approach, view, statement, or opinion of the author(s) or producer(s), which may be helpful to others who face similar situations.

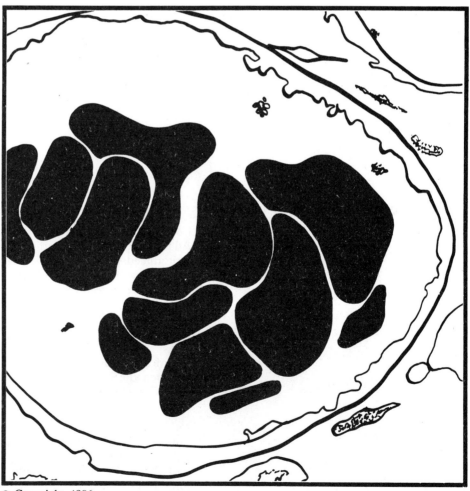

© Copyright, 1986
American Academy of Orthopaedic Surgeons

Editorial Board

Medical Illustration

Credits

Book Design: Swiss Graphics, Chicago
Photography: James Koepfler, Boston
Typesetting: Total Typography, Chicago
Printing: Banta-Harrisonburg (Virginia division)

First Edition

Library of Congress Cataloging in Publication Data

American Academy of Orthopaedic Surgeons
Orthopaedic Science
ISBN O-89203-011-9

Published by The American Academy of Orthopaedic Surgeons
222 South Prospect Avenue
Park Ridge, Illinois 60068-4058
June, 1986

Sheldon R. Simon, M.D., Project Director
Richard S. Riggins, M.D., Chairman,
    Committee on Basic Sciences
Carl R. Wirth, M.D., Local Arrangements

Jonathan Black, Ph.D

Adele L. Boskey, Ph.D.

Carl T. Brighton, M.D., Ph.D.

Joseph A. Buckwalter, M.D.

Albert H. Burstein, Ph.D.

William K. Dunham, M.D.

Robert H. Fitzgerald, Jr., M.D.

Victor M. Goldberg, M.D.

Wilson C. Hayes, Ph.D.

James H. Herndon, M.D.

John D. Hsu, M.D.

Frederick S. Kaplan, M.D.

Joseph M. Lane, M.D.

Jerry Maynard, M.D.

Van C. Mow, Ph.D.

Alan L. Schiller, M.D.

Myron Spector, Ph.D.

Dempsey Springfield, M.D.

Savio L-Y Woo, Ph.D

Timothy M. Wright, M.D.

Committee on Basic Sciences

Richard S. Riggins, M.D., Chairman

Roy K. Aaron, M.D.
Carl T. Brighton, M.D., Consultant
John L. Eady, M.D.
Melvin J. Glimcher, M.D.
R. Bruce Heppenstall, M.D.
John D. Hsu, M.D.
Joseph M. Lane, M.D., Consultant
Thomas A. Lange, M.D.
Michael A. Simon, M.D.
Sheldon R. Simon, M.D.
Carl R. Wirth, M.D.

Contributors

Basic Science Seminars 1977-1984

Orthopaedic Science: A Resource and Self-Study Guide for the Practitioner is based on presentations at basic science seminars sponsored by the Academy from 1977-1984. Persons giving presentations at these seminars include the following:

Stephen Abrahamson, Ph.D. (1978)

Wayne H. Akeson, M.D. (1977, 1980, 1981, 1984)

James A. Albright, M.D. (1984)

David Amiel, M.S. (1981)

H. C. Amstutz, M.D. (1977)

Steven P. Arnoczky, D.V.M., Dipl. ACVS, (1984)

Rodney K. Beals, M.D. (1978)

Jonathan Black, Ph.D. (1977, 1984)

J. David Blaha, M.D. (1984)

Henry H. Bohlman, M.D. (1983)

B. Kaye Boles, Ph.D. (1981)

Robert E. Booth, Jr., M.D. (1981)

Adele L. Boskey, Ph.D. (1980)

Richard A. Brand, M.D. (1983)

H. Robert Brashear, M.D. (1977)

Carl T. Brighton, M.D., Ph.D. (1977, 1978, 1981, 1983)

Stanley A. Brown, D. Eng. (1984)

Joseph A. Buckwalter, M.S., M.D. (1983, 1984)

Peter G. Bullough, M.D. (1980)

Albert H. Burstein, Ph.D. (1978)

Peter H. Byers, M.D. (1983)

Dennis R. Carter, Ph.D. (1980, 1983)

Ted A. Chaglassian, M.D. (1980)

Edmund Y.S. Chao (1980, 1983, 1984)

F. Richard Convery, M.D. (1981)

Reginald R. Cooper, M.D. (1977)

Richard L. Cruess, M.D. (1977)

Hector F. DeLuca, Ph.D. (1977)

James G. Dillon, Ph.D. (1984)

Howard D. Dorfman, M.D. (1978)

Frederick R. Eilber, M.D. (1978)

Harvard Ellman, M.D. (1983)

Charles H. Epps, Jr., M.D. (1980)

Michael Erlich, M.D. (1983)

C. McCollister Evarts, M.D. (1980)

David Eyre, Ph.D. (1978, 1981)

Gerald Finerman, M.D. (1978, 1980, 1983)

Robert H. Fitzgerald, M.D. (1980)

Steven R. Garfin, M.D. (1981)

Richard H. Gelberman, M.D. (1984)

Melvin J. Glimcher, M.D. (1981)

Amy Beth Goldman, M.D. (1981)

Philip D. Gollnick, Ph.D. (1981)

A. Seth Greenwald, Ph.D. (1977)

Allan E. Gross, M.D., F.R.C.S. (1981)

Gary R. Grotendorst, Ph.D. (1984)

Jose Guerra, M.D. (1981)

Wilson C. Hayes, Ph.D. (1980)

Anthony K. Hedley, M.D. (1983)

James H. Herndon, M.D. (1980)

David S. Hungerford, M.D. (1983)

James M. Hunter, M.D. (1980)

Sergio A. Jimenez, M.D. (1981)

James O. Johnston, M.D. (1977, 1983)

Peter Jokl, M.D. (1980)

Jenifer Jowsey, Ph.D. (1978, 1980)

Herbert Kaufer, M.D. (1977)

Patrick J. Kelly, M.D. (1977, 1978, 1980, 1981)

Peter T. Kirchner, M.D. (1981)

David R. Knighton, M.D. (1984)

William Krause, Ph.D. (1984)

Eugene M. Lance, M.D., Ph.D. (1981)

Joseph M. Lane, M.D. (1977, 1978, 1981, 1983)

Eugene P. Lautenschlager, Ph.D. (1978)

Stephen J. Lipson, M.D. (1981)

Goran Lundborg, M.D., Ph.D. (1981)

Arthur F. Mak, Ph.D. (1983)

John Makley, M.D. (1978)

Henry J. Mankin, M.D. (1978)

Roger Mann, M.D. (1981)

Keith Markolf, Ph.D. (1978, 1983)

Mary-Blair Matejczyk, M.D. (1977)

Frederick A. Matsen, III, M.D. (1981)

John Matyas, B.A. (1984)

Jerry Maynard, Ph.D. (1978, 1980)

Allen Meisel, M.D. (1980)

Katharine Merritt, Ph.D. (1984)

Introduction

The continuing interest of the Academy in basic science concepts important to the practice of orthopaedics has led to this volume, an attempt to assemble in one place many of the essentials of orthopaedic science. Over the years, the Academy has sponsored workshops for basic science educators in orthopaedics. At each of these sessions, orthopaedists and researchers made presentations on a variety of subjects, with the end result being the exchange of the latest knowledge and the production of material to be used in teaching orthopaedic science.

From these workshops, six syllabi and more than 7500 color slides were produced, an enormous amount of information that represented considerable time and study. As the number of these syllabi and slide sets grew and rapid advances in orthopaedic science occurred, it became clear to the Academy's Committee on Basic Sciences that a concerted effort to consolidate, update, and organize this massive amount of information was necessary. The goal was to present a body of information that would be helpful to all clinicians interested in basic science.

In January, 1985, the committee, under the chairmanship of Carl T. Brighton, M.D., proposed to the Academy's Board of Directors that the Academy sponsor this project. As part of this effort, a special workshop would be held to review the existing slide sets and accompanying syllabi and thus determine what available material as well as new material best represented orthopaedic science. The Academy's board accepted the proposal and provided major funding for the project.

A select group of orthopaedists and basic scientists representing each area of musculoskeletal basic science met in Mohonk, N.Y., in September, 1985. Beth Ingraham, medical illustrator for the project, was also present to make preliminary sketches for new slides and illustrations. Karen Schneider of the Academy staff provided valuable assistance in coordinating the five-day meeting.

The material reviewed and produced at the workshop had to be edited, compiled, and put in a format appropriate for all those interested in orthopaedic science. This assignment was carried out by a small group of individuals from the Committee on Basic Sciences: Sheldon R. Simon, M.D., Project Director, Richard S. Riggins, M.D., and Carl R. Wirth, M.D. Ably assisting the group, especially in text editing and project coordination, was the Academy's Senior Medical Editor, Marilyn Fox, Ph.D.

After reviewing the text and slides produced and selected at the Mohonk workshop, it was decided that a significant number of new slides should be created. In addition, the editorial committee decided to include in the syllabus a line illustration corresponding to each one of the slides. These illustrations would highlight the most important aspects of the slides and also ensure that the syllabus could be used as a self-study guide. This has been done, working very closely with the medical illustrator. Thus, while the ideal way to study the material is to review the syllabus and the slides together, it is hoped that the illustrated syllabus can also communicate the essence of the material.

All attempts have been made to ensure that the syllabus and slides fulfill the educational purposes intended. The editorial committee recognizes that certain topics are not covered as extensively as they might have been. Furthermore, the syllabus represents standard knowledge in the field, and as such includes little material and information of a speculative or experimental nature.

In this project there are many people to thank: those involved in the original scientific presentations, the Mohonk workshop, the text editing, the illustration work, and the organizational details of mounting what has become a major investment by the Academy. The contributors list on the preceding pages notes all of those who made presentations at the basic science workshops held between 1977 and 1984, as well as those who participated at Mohonk. Their participation and contribution of ideas, material, and most of all their time are all greatly appreciated. In addition to the Academy staff members mentioned above, staff members who contributed to this project include Mark W. Wieting, Director of Communications and Publications, Catherine Smith, Alice Michaels, and Geri Dubberke. Finally, Nancy Davis from Dr. Simon's staff, Barbara Smith and Gayle Michael from Dr. Riggins' staff, and Peggy Pulfer from Dr. Wirth's staff deserve thanks for accomplishing the initial word processing of the text and managing other details.

The Committee on Basic Sciences hopes the syllabus and slides will prove to be a valuable teaching tool in the science of orthopaedics. We invite your comments and suggestions for improving it, and can be reached through the Academy's office in Park Ridge, Illinois.

Table of Contents

VI   Biomaterials

VII   Non-skeletal Disorders Complicating Orthopaedic Practice

VIII   Illustration and Slide Index

IX   Subject Index

Chapter I

Anatomy

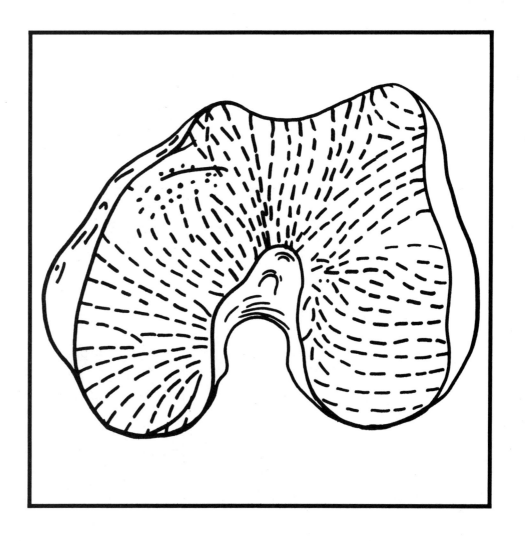

This chapter will discuss basic anatomical concepts relating to bone, cartilage, muscle, tendon and nerve in order to enhance the discussion of disease processes and material properties of human tissue presented in later chapters. Where possible, each section will relate the information presented to clinical situations.

Structure and Composition of Bone

Bone is amazingly well organized at all levels from the molecular to the gross. Its arrangement provides a tensile strength nearly that of cast iron, but with great economy of material and relatively little weight. As Slide I,1 illustrates, at the microscopic or material level bone consists of two forms; woven bone and lamellar bone. Woven bone is considered immature bone, or primitive bone, and is found in the embryo and the newborn, in fracture callus and the metaphyseal region of growing bone.

Woven bone, or primary bone, is coarse-fibered and contains no uniform orientation of collagen fibrils. It has more cells per unit volume than does lamellar bone. Its mineral content varies and its cells are randomly arranged. The relatively disoriented collagen fibers of woven bone give it isotropic mechanical characteristics; i.e., when tested, the mechanical behavior of woven bone is similar regardless of the orientation of the applied forces.

One month after birth, lamellar bone begins to form. By one year of age it is actively replacing woven bone, as the latter is resorbed. By age four, most normal bone is lamellar bone. It is, therefore, a more mature bone resulting from the remodeling of woven or previously existing bone. Lamellar bone is found in several structural and functional systems: trabecular lamellae; outer and inner circumferential lamellae; interstitial lamellae; and osteons with concentric lamellae. The well-organized, stress-oriented collagen of lamellar bone imparts anisotropic properties to bone; i.e., the mechanical behavior of bone is different depending on the orientation of the applied forces.

As also illustrated in Slide I,1, woven bone and lamellar bone are structurally organized into *trabecular* (spongy or cancellous) bone and *cortical* (dense or compact) bone. (*Plexiform* bone and *haversian* bone are two types of compact bone.)

Trabecular bone is found at the ends of long bones near the joints and in cuboid bones such as the vertebrae. The internal beams or spicules of trabecular bone form a three-dimensional branching lattice work aligned along areas of stress. Trabecular bone is subjected mainly to compressive forces. Slide I,2 illustrates new woven bone in a trabecular pattern with no discernible matrix orientation (left panel) compared to the layered arrangement of matrix fibers in lamellar bone arranged in a trabecular pattern (right panel).

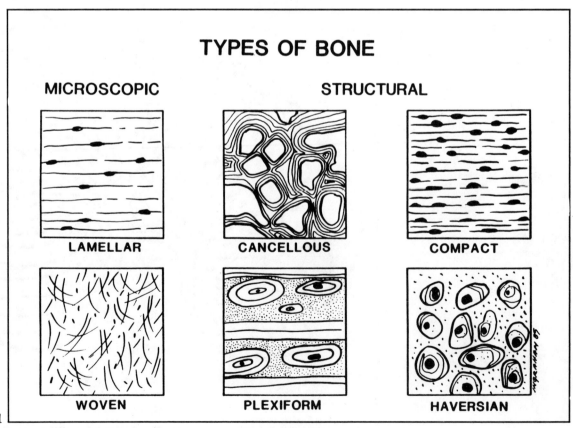

TYPES OF BONE

MICROSCOPIC **STRUCTURAL**

LAMELLAR CANCELLOUS COMPACT

WOVEN PLEXIFORM HAVERSIAN

Slide I,1

Cortical bone is found in cuboid and long bones. Cortical bone is subject to bending and torsional forces as well as to compressive forces. In small animals there is no special arrangement of the vascular network in cortical bone; it consists simply of layers of lamellar bone, called compact bone. In larger animals that experience rapid growth, cortical bone is made up of layers of lamellar bone and woven bone, with the vascular channels located mainly in the woven bone. This bone is termed plexiform bone. (See Slide I,1.) Such an arrangement of bone allows rapid growth and the accumulation of large amounts of bone over a short time.

Haversian bone is probably the most complex type of cortical bone. It is composed of vascular channels circumferentially surrounded by lamellar bone. This com-plex arrangement of bone around the vascular channel is called the *osteon*. Named by Biederman in 1914, it is an irregular, branching and anastomosing cylinder composed of a more or less centrally placed neurovascular canal surrounded by cell-permeated layers of bone matrix. Osteons are usually oriented in the long axis of the bone and are the major structural units of cortical bone. Cortical bone is, therefore, a complex of many adjacent osteons and their interstitial and circumferential lamellae. Slide I,3 illustrates a single osteon surrounded by interstitial lamellae. Slide I,4 shows a photomicrograph of cortical bone from a femoral shaft with inner circumferential lamellae next to the marrow cavity (lower left corner). Also shown are many osteons with their concentric lamellae, and the interstitial lamellae between osteons.

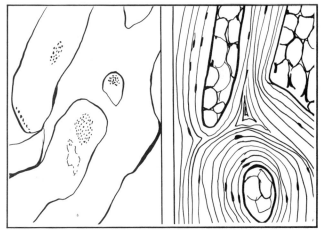

Slide I,2

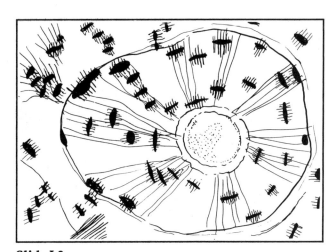

Slide I,3

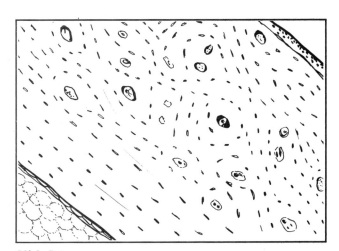

Slide I,4

The central canal of an osteon, called the haversian canal, contains cells, vessels and occasionally nerves. Most vessels in the haversian canals have the ultrastructural features of capillaries, although some smaller-sized vessels may resemble lymphatic vessels. Slide I,5 is an electron photomicrograph of a large capillary containing red cells in a haversian canal. Adjacent to it is a smaller vessel containing only precipitated protein; its endothelial wall is not surrounded by a basement membrane. Such features are characteristic of lymphatic vessels. The basement membrane of capillary walls may function as a rate-limiting or selective ion-limiting transport barrier, since all material traversing the vessel wall must go through the basement membrane. The presence of this barrier is of particular importance regarding calcium and phosphorus ion transport to and from bone.

The capillaries in the central canals are derived from the principal nutrient arteries of the bone or the epiphyseal-metaphyseal arteries. Slide I,6 (left panel) shows the nutrient artery of a long bone entering the shaft and branching to form the vascular network in cortical bone. By using lower magnification and injecting India ink (right panel), the complexity of this vascular network is better shown.

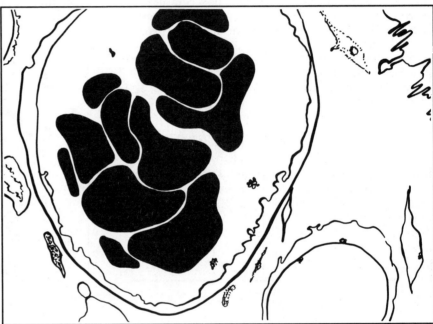

Slide I,5

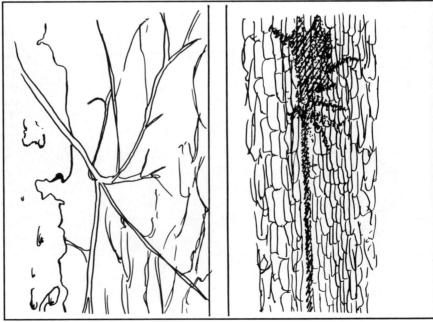

Slide I,6

Bone Cells

Osteoblasts The major types of bone cells are the osteoblasts, osteocytes, and osteoclasts. Osteoblasts are best seen wherever new bone matrix is forming. Slide I,7 shows light and electron photomicrographs of osteoblasts adjacent to new bone. By light microscopy (left panel), some osteoblasts appear rectangular with their long axes perpendicular to the osteoid or bone surface. They seem to be polarized, with the basophilic cytoplasm near the bone and the nucleus at the end of the cell away from the bone surface. Osteoblasts contain an abundance of rough-surfaced endoplasmic reticulum, a characteristic of cells that manufacture protein for export from the cell (right panel). In addition to an extensive endoplasmic reticulum, osteoblasts contain a well-developed golgi apparatus and numerous mitochondria. Histochemical studies have demonstrated that alkaline phosphatase is distributed over the outer surface of the osteoblast cell membrane. As indicated by the electron photomicrograph, there is a layer of newly formed bone (osteoid) between the osteoblast cell membrane and the mineralized matrix of older bone.

Osteocytes Once an osteoblast becomes surrounded by bone matrix, which then becomes mineralized, the cell is characterized by a higher nucleus-to-cytoplasm ratio and contains fewer organelles. Such a cell is the osteocyte of bone, and although osteocytes are the most numerous of bone cells they seem to receive the least amount of attention. Light microscopy (Slide I,3) reveals osteocytes arranged concentrically around the lumen of an osteon. Their canaliculi radiate as striae parallel to the radii of the osteon. Cells lie in and between lamellae. Osteocyte lacunae are uniformly oriented with respect to the longitudinal and radial axes of lamellae. Osteoblasts and osteocytes have extensive cell processes which project through the canaliculi, thereby establishing contact between adjacent osteocytes and the central canals of osteons. Slide I,8 illustrates an electron photomicrograph of a mature osteocyte with its decreased organelle content, greater nucleus-to-cytoplasm ratio, and numerous cell processes extending outward through the canaliculi.

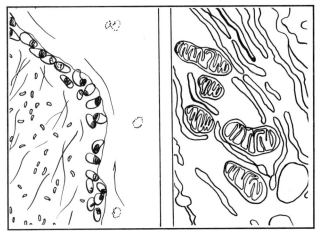

Slide I,7

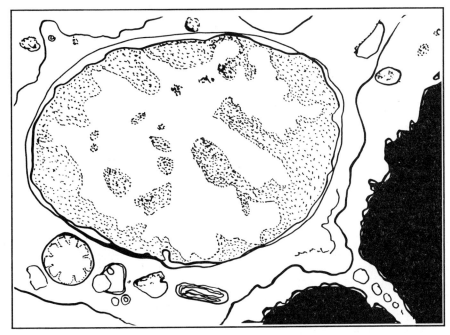

Slide I,8

Osteocytes can metabolically manipulate their environment more or less independent of surface resorption and accretion. This ability is important to cellular regulation of calcium exchange. Bone crystals are extremely small and have a surface area of approximately 100 m²/g or a total of 100 acres of surface area in the adult human body. Most of these crystals, buried away from the endosteal and periosteal bone surfaces, appear to be unavailable to effect the necessary exchange with extracellular fluid, making it difficult to explain the immediate exchange of bone mineral with the extracellular fluid. There is, however, a vast surface area on the haversian canal and lacunar walls and an even larger area on the canalicular walls, which in the adult totals about 3000 m², or 3 acres where bone mineral exchange with extracellular fluid can take place.

Osteoclasts Osteoclasts are the major resorptive cells of bone and are characterized by multiple nuclei. Osteoclasts are derived from pleuripotential cells of the bone marrow. Early research on osteopetrosis using rodent models revealed that reversal of the disease occurred with successful bone marrow allografts. Recent clinical trials demonstrated new osteoclast populations in patients receiving successful bone marrow allografts.

As illustrated in Slide I,9, osteoclasts lie in regions of bone resorption in pits called Howship's lacunae. The electron photomicrograph in I,9 (right panel) demonstrates a paucity of rough-surfaced endoplasmic reticulum, a moderate number of ribosomes, numerous smooth vesicles, and well-developed mitochondria. As shown in the histologic section of Slide I,9, the other major feature of the osteoclast is the brush border, which results from extensive infoldings of the cell membrane adjacent to the resorptive surface. Osteoclasts appearing some distance from the surface of bone do not have brush borders and are called "inactive" or "resting" osteoclasts. Direct observations show that the brush border of the osteoclast sweeps across the surface of bone. The infolding of the brush border greatly increases the surface area of the plasma membrane. This structural feature appears only over disrupted bone surfaces. The infolds of the brush border end in numerous channels and vesicles in the cell cytoplasm. Within these channels and vesicles lie numerous mineral crystals.

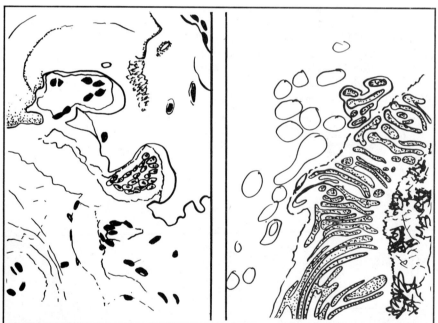

Slide I,9

Mineralization

Mineralization of skeletal tissues can be considered as having two distinct phases: first, formation of the initial mineral deposit (initiation); and second, proliferation or accretion of additional mineral crystals on these initial mineral deposits (growth). Of the total body mineral, only a small percentage is thought to represent the initial deposit. The bulk of the mineral comes from growth of the initial crystalline material.

Initiation of mineralization requires a combination of events, including increases in the local concentration of precipitating ions, formation or exposure of mineral nucleators, and removal or modification of mineralization inhibitors. The vast majority of mineral in the body is an analogue of the naturally occurring mineral, hydroxyapatite, shown in Slide I,10. The hydroxyapatite in bone is extremely small (200 to 400 angstroms in largest dimension) and contains numerous impurities, adsorbed onto the surface, or incorporated within the crystal. The increased solubility of bone mineral crystals, relative to geological mineral or crystals in tooth enamel, is due to both crystal size and the impurities. It must be noted that the nature of the first mineral crystals deposited is still unknown. Extracellular matrix vesicles, located at a distance from the collagen fibrils, have been identified as the site of initial mineral deposition in young, calcifying cartilage and in young bone.

More energy is required to form the initial mineral crystals than is required to add ions or ion clusters to already existing crystals. Secondary nucleation, the growth of small crystallites in a branching manner from the surface of other small crystals, also requires less energy than does *de novo* initiation. To circumvent the large energy required of initial hydroxyapatite formation, a less stable (or metastable) precursor phase may form first, and later be either converted directly to hydroxyapatite or serve as a heterogeneous nucleator of hydroxyapatite. Once primary nucleation has occurred, there is an early rapid increase in size from "crystal nuclei" to the first solid phase particles initially observed by electron microscopy. This proces is termed "crystal growth." Operationally we have defined the two processes of primary nucleation and crystal growth as *multiplication.*

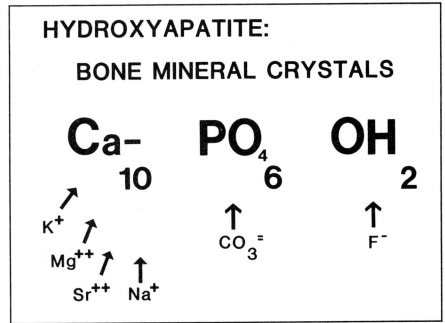

Slide I,10

Collagen forms about 96% of unmineralized bone matrix. The rest consists of a small amount of proteoglycan and noncollagenous proteins. Since the final appearance of lamellae probably reflects the initial orientation of collagen, it is important to examine the arrangement of these fibrils in unmineralized matrix, as illustrated in Slide I,11. Centrally in the haversian canal, collagen fibrils arrange themselves rather poorly. However, at the periphery, they organize in definite 1-to-3 micron layers, with the long axes of collagen fibrils oriented in different directions in adjacent lamellae.

Of the connective tissue collagens, only type I (bone, tendon, skin) collagen can accept hydroxyapatite deposition *in vitro*. It has been shown that mineralized type I collagen contains crosslinks that are chemically different from those in nonmineralized osteoid. Such collagen crosslinking may also affect the distribution of mineral within the collagen. We do not know what causes the orientation of matrix fibrils in lamellae; however, the pattern obviously forms prior to mineralization.

Petruska and Hodge postulated a quarter stagger theory of macromolecular aggregation for collagen wherein adjacent tropocollagen molecules overlap, leaving a space between the ends of the molecules, the so-called hole zones in the collagen fibrils. There are also "pores" between adjacent macromolecules.

Collagen intraperiod bands are located at the loci of amino acid polar side chains on adjacent tropocollagen molecules. These bands span about 400 angstroms and each have a 670-angstrom period. The mineral exhibits a definite relationship to intraperiod bands. Mineral deposition seems to start at the fibril edge and spread into the interior. The region of mineral infiltration corresponds to the "hole zones" in the Petruska-Hodge model.

Some noncollagenous proteins, such as the phosphoproteins and osteonectin-collagen complexes, seem to promote collagen mineralization. In addition, certain proteolipids and calcium acidic-phospholipid phosphate complexes also seem to promote hydroxyapatite deposition *in vitro*. Extracellular matrix vesicles may facilitate calcification by (1) concentrating ions, (2) providing a protective environment free of mineralization inhibitors, or (3) providing enzymes involved in matrix modification.

Slide I,12 shows that initial mineral deposition may be promoted both by the formation or exposure of nucleators and by the removal or modification of inhibitors. *In vitro* proteoglycans extracted from both calcifying and noncalcifying cartilage inhibit hydroxyapatite growth. Initial mineralization of collagen is a process that is still being investigated intensely.

Secondary nucleation After deposition of amorphous calcium phosphate into collagen (mineral nucleation of osteoid), more and more hydroxyapatite must be added to give bone its rigidity. While some of the new mineral added to osteoid is deposited by initial nucleation, most of the additional mineral is acquired by a process known as secondary nucleation, in which new crystals of apatite are deposited on nuclei of hydroxyapatite already contained within the holes and pores of the osteoid. This accretion of new mineral continues until bone is fully mineralized.

In summary, from the physical-chemical standpoint, mineral accretion *in tissues* arises by (1) primary or heterogenous nucleation; (2) crystal growth; and (3) secondary nucleation induced by previously formed crystals.

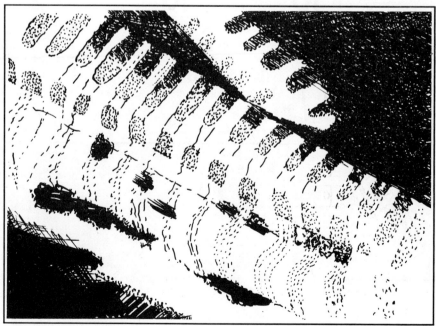

Slide I,11

Correlation between biological and physical-chemical heterogeneity The increase in the number of mineral phase particles in the collagen fibrils that accompanies mineral accretion can, of course, occur either in the holes or pores, as depicted in Slide I,13. From the spatial point of view, calcification even at the level of the electron microscope reveals that mineralization proceeds as a *discontinuous process*. Discrete, physically separated loci within the osteoid fibrils become impregnated with mineral particles about the same time, forming a number of mineralization sites. It appears that simultaneously but at different locations within collagen fibrils, initial mineralization takes place. Electron microscopy indicates that as crystal growth and secondary nucleation continue, the discrete growth areas enlarge and eventually coalesce. An understanding of how mineral accretion in bone as a whole proceeds once nucleation begins in any one compartment will become important during discussions of the influence of various metabolic and nutritional diseases upon bone mineralization.

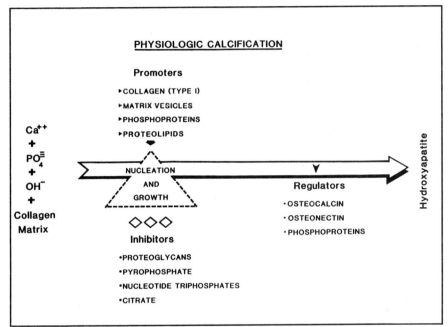

Slide I,12

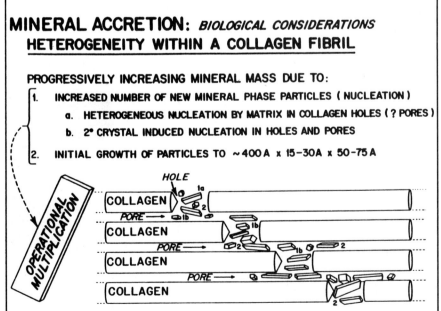

Slide I,13

Bone Development

Slide I,14 demonstrates typical endochondral bone development. The human long bone begins in early embryonic life as a cartilaginous anlage of the future bone. In the human long bone, cartilage cells in the central portion of the anlage enlarge and become hypertrophic, and the surrounding matrix becomes calcified (Slide I,14B). About the same time, a bone collar forms around the periphery. This collar is the first bone formed and is an example of mesenchymal bone formation.

At the beginning of fetal life, a vascular invasion occurs through the bone collar into the central portion of the bone (Slide I,14C). The vascular cells lay down a nidus of bone on the previously calcified cartilage. This process is termed endochondral bone formation. This nidus is the primary center of ossification and grows centrifugally toward each end of the bone Slide (I,14D). At a rather definite time, a secondary center of ossification appears (Slide I,14E) and is termed the epiphysis. It likewise grows and expands centrifugally in all directions, although at a much slower rate than the primary ossification center. As the distance between the bone growing in the primary

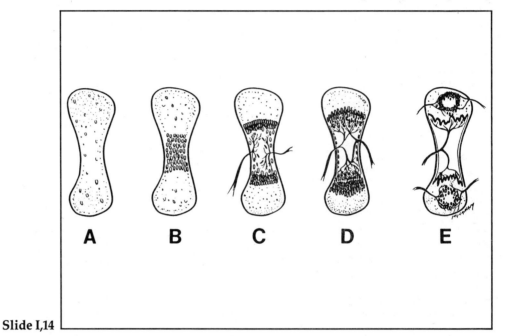

Slide I,14

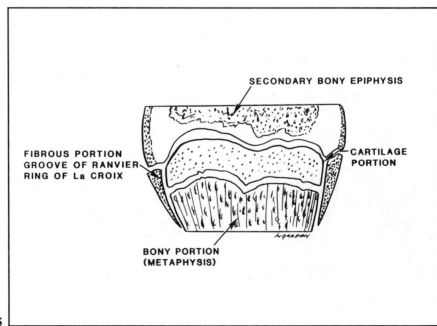

Slide I,15

ossification center and epiphysis gradually decreases, the portion of the epiphysis that faces the primary ossification center closes and becomes sealed with condensed bone, termed the bone plate. The cartilage trapped between the two ossification centers is termed the growth plate, or physis.

As illustrated in I,15, the physis consists of a cartilaginous component, itself divided into various histologic zones; a bony component, or metaphysis; and a fibrous component surrounding the periphery of the plate, consisting of a wedge-shaped groove of cells termed the groove of Ranvier and a ring of fibrous tissue and bone termed the perichondrial ring of LaCroix. While the ossification groove and the perichondrial ring are part of the same structure, they have different functions. The function of the groove of Ranvier is to provide chondrocytes for circumferential growth, while the perichondrial ring acts as a limiting membrane mechanically supporting the growth plate.

As noted in Slide I,16, each of the three components of the growth plate has its own distinct blood supply. The epiphyseal artery supplies the epiphysis. The metaphysis is richly supplied with blood both from terminal branches of the nutrient artery and from the metaphyseal arteries. The nutrient artery supplies the central 80% of the metaphysis, whereas the metaphyseal vessels supply only the peripheral regions. Terminal branches from each of these arteries pass vertically toward the physis and end in vascular loops at the base of physis. The vessels turn back at this level, eventually drawing into the large central vein of the diaphysis. All or most of the vascular loops are closed. The fibrous peripheral structures of the growth plate, the groove of Ranvier and the perichondrial ring of LaCroix are richly supplied with blood.

The cartilaginous portion of the growth plate is divided into various zones according to morphology or function. As shown in Slide I,17, these include the reserve zone, the proliferative zone and the hypertrophic zone. Only the proliferative zone of the cartilage is supplied with blood. The hypertrophic zone is entirely avascular. This fact has important implications concerning chondrocyte metabolism and matrix calcification.

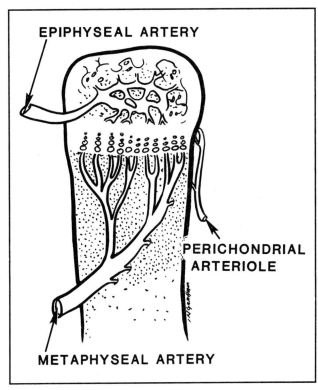

EPIPHYSEAL ARTERY

PERICHONDRIAL ARTERIOLE

METAPHYSEAL ARTERY

Slide I,16

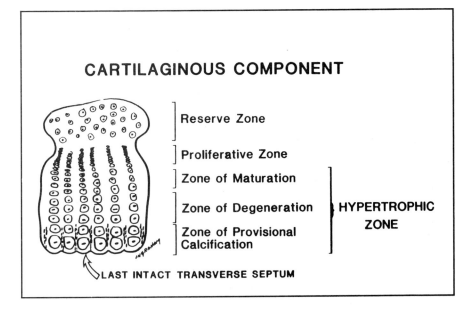

CARTILAGINOUS COMPONENT

Reserve Zone

Proliferative Zone

Zone of Maturation

Zone of Degeneration

Zone of Provisional Calcification

HYPERTROPHIC ZONE

LAST INTACT TRANSVERSE SEPTUM

Slide I,17

In the reserve zone the cells appear to be storing lipids and other materials, reserving them for later nutritional requirements. The cytoplasm of these cells contains glycogen and an abundant endoplasmic reticulum, the latter indicating active protein synthesis. The reserve zone contains more hydroxyproline than any zone in the plate, as well as neutral polysaccharide, or aggregated proteoglycan. Blood passes through the reserve zone in cartilage canals to arborize at the top of the proliferative zone, resulting in low oxygen tension in the reserve zone.

The function of the proliferative zone is twofold: (1) matrix production, and (2) cellular proliferation. These two functions produce longitudinal growth. Chondrocytes in the reserve zone give way to flattened chondrocytes in the proliferative zone aligned in longitudinal columns. The cytoplasm of these cells still contains glycogen and endoplasmic reticulum. The relatively high oxygen tension in the proliferative zone, coupled with the presence of glycogen in the chondrocytes, demonstrates aerobic metabolism. Chondrocytes are the only cells in the cartilaginous portion of the growth plate that divide. The top cell of each column is the true "mother" cell and is the true germinal layer of the growth plate.

The matrix of the proliferative zone contains randomly distributed collagen fibrils, matrix vesicles, neutral glycoproteins, and proteoglycan aggregates. Oxygen tension is higher in the proliferative zone than in any other zone of the growth plate because of the rich vascular supply present at the top of the zone.

The functions of the hypertrophic zone seem clear: (1) to prepare the matrix for calcification, and (2) to calcify the matrix. In the hypertrophic zone, the chondrocytes become spherical and greatly enlarged. From the top to the bottom of the proliferative zone, the chondrocytes swell and progressively lose their cytoplasmic organelles and glycogen content. The average chondrocyte in the hypertrophic zone is five times larger than the average chondrocyte in the proliferative zone. The cells appear dead or dying.

Histochemical localization of calcium in the hypertrophic zone gives some clues as to how mineralization of the cartilaginous columns takes place. The upper left electron photomicrograph of Slide I,18 shows a conventionally stained mitochondrion. The upper right frame shows the mitochondrion stained for calcium. The lower right frame shows a mitochondrion in the top of the hypertrophic zone stained for calcium. Note the loss of calcium toward the bottom of the zone (lower left frame). Thus, Slide I,18 illustrates that mitochondrial calcium is progressively lost from the top to the bottom of the hypertrophic zone. The calcium lost may be involved in cartilage matrix mineralization.

Slide I,19 summarizes the metabolic events occurring in the growth plate. In the proliferative zone, oxygen tension is high, aerobic metabolism occurs, glycogen is stored, and mitochondria form ATP. Mitochondria can form ATP or store calcium, but both processes cannot occur simultaneously. In the proliferative zone, the energy requirement for matrix production and cellular proliferation is high, the mitochondria form ATP but do not store calcium. In the hypertrophic zone, oxygen tension is low, anaerobic metabolism occurs, and glycogen is consumed. In the top portion of the hypertrophic zone, mitochondria switch from forming ATP to accumulating calcium. In the bottom half of the hypertrophic zone, glycogen is depleted. In this area of low oxygen tension, there is no other source of nutrition for energy. The cells die, and the mitochondria give up their calcium.

Slide I,20 shows a growth plate stained with PAS/Alcian blue. Near the top of the slide is the red matrix of the reserve and proliferating zones, representing neutral glycoproteins and proteoglycan aggregates. The red stain gives way to a blue-stained matrix in the hypertrophic zone, which represents acid glycoproteins and disaggregated proteoglycans.

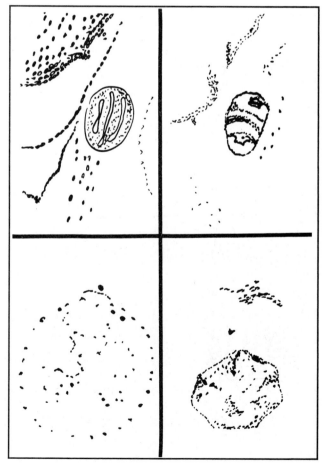

Slide I,18

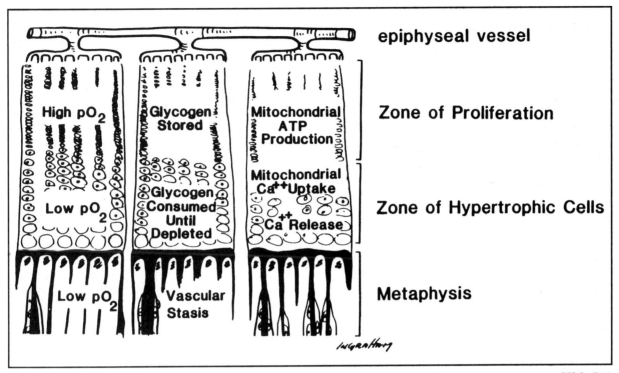

epiphyseal vessel

Zone of Proliferation

Zone of Hypertrophic Cells

Metaphysis

Slide I,19

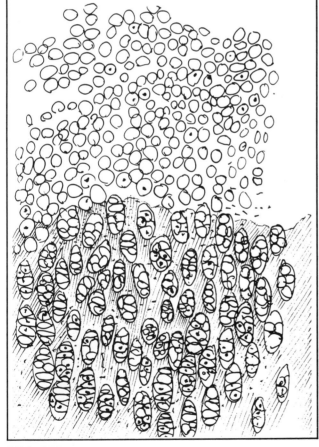

Slide I,20

Slide I,21 illustrates the progressive decrease in the number of subunits of the proteoglycan aggregates from the reserve zone through the zone of provisional calcification in the hypertrophic zone. The distance between the subunits increases as well. It is believed the large, tightly packed subunits of the reserve and hypertrophic zones may inhibit mineralization, whereas smaller aggregates with widely spaced subunits at the bottom of the hypertrophic zone may be less effective in preventing mineral growth. Degradation of proteoglycan aggregates takes place before significant mineralization of the cartilage in the growth plate occurs.

Slide I,22 is an electron photomicrograph of four matrix vesicles. They are very small structures, measuring 1000 to 1500 angstroms in diameter and enclosed in a trilamellar membrane produced by the chondrocyte. Matrix vesicles are rich in alkaline phosphatase, a pyrophosphatase that can destroy pyrophosphate, another inhibitor of calcium phosphate precipitation. Slide I,22 depicts the vesicles at various stages of calcification. The initial calcification, called "seeding or nucleation" that occurs in the growth plate in the bottom of the hypertrophic zone does so within or upon matrix vesicles present in the longitudinal septa of the matrix.

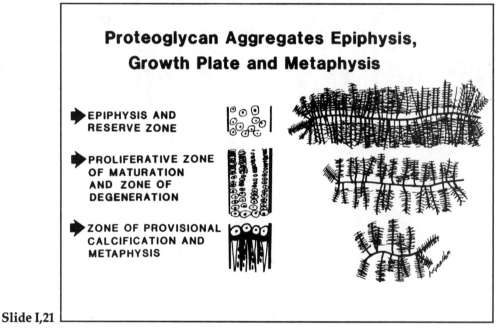

Slide I,21

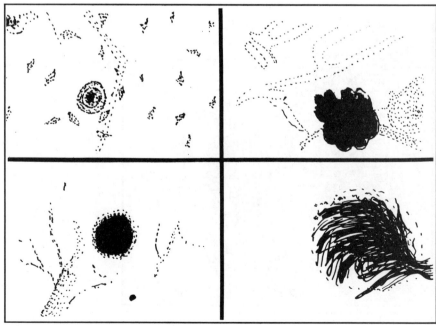

Slide I,22

With crystal growth and confluence, the longitudinal septa become calcified. This process occurs in the bottom portion of the hypertrophic zone in a region frequently called the zone of provisional calcification. Calcification of this section makes the intercellular matrix of the section relatively impermeable to metabolites. Slide I,23 summarizes the process of cartilage mineralization. As calcification occurs diffusion of nutrients and oxygen to the hypertrophic chondrocyte is decreased, anaerobic glycolysis with glycogen consumption occurs until all the glycogen is depleted, mitochondria release calcium, nucleation occurs in the matrix vesicles, and crystal growth and confluence mineralizes the longitudinal septa. Thus, a cycle is established that ultimately results in the death of the hypertrophic chondrocyte and mineralization of the cartilage.

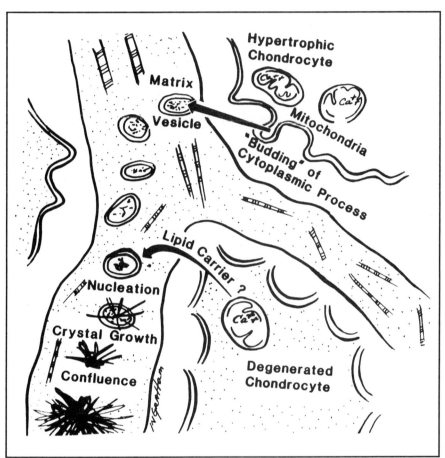

Slide I,23

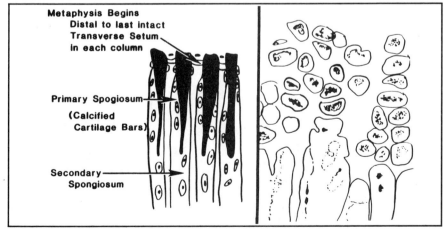

Slide I,24

Slide I,24 is a composite slide showing a diagram and photomicrograph of the beginning portions of the metaphysis. The functions of the metaphysis are as follows: (1) vascular invasion of the transverse septa at the bottom of the cartilaginous portion of the growth plate; (2) bone formation; (3) material remodeling of calcified cartilage bars and replacement of fiber bone with lamellar bone; and (4) structural remodeling, or funnelization of the metaphysis.

The metaphysis begins just distal to the last intact transverse septum at the base of each cell column of the cartilage portion of the growth plate. The metaphysis ends in the region where narrowing or funnelization of the bone end ceases.

Capillary loops of endothelial and perivascular cells invade the base of the cartilaginous portion of the plate. Cytoplasmic processes from these cells push into the transverse septa and remove the nonmineralized matrix. At this same level in the metaphysis, the longitudinal septa are partially or completely calcified. Osteoblasts line the calcified longitudinal septa. This region in the metaphysis with little bone formation is termed the primary spongiosum. The secondary spongiosum begins in the region where the osteoblasts initiate endochondral bone formation on the calcified longitudinal septa. Osteoclasts are seen evenly distributed throughout the entire metaphysis, except in the primary spongiosum. Still farther down in the metaphysis, the fiber bone originally formed is replaced with lamellar bone. This gradual replacement of the calcified longitudinal septa with newly formed fiber bone, as well as the gradual replacement of fiber bone with lamellar bone, is termed internal remodeling. Osteoclasts subperiosteally located around the outside of the metaphysis participate in external remodeling. Encircling the growth plate are the ossification groove of Ranvier and the perichondrial ring of LaCroix. These structures are shown in Slide I,25.

Growth Plate Abnormalities

Many abnormalities of the growth plate exist. The study of such abnormalities is severely restricted due to the lack of available tissue for analysis. For this reason, and for the sake of brevity, only four growth plate abnormalities will be presented here, each an example taken from a different part of the plate.

Achondroplasia Achondroplasia is an autosomal dominant disease in which endochondral bone formation is severely inhibited, but membranous bone formation is normal. The basic defect may be an inability to carry on oxidative phosphorylation at normal rates. Slide I,26 shows the typical histologic and radiographic appearance of this disorder. The primary defect in the growth plate is in the proliferative zone where chondrocyte proliferation is decreased, cells are scanty, and column formation is poor or does not occur at all. The lack of chondrocyte proliferation and the subsequent scanty matrix production result in decreased longitudinal growth. Subperiosteal membranous bone formation is normal, so the width of the shaft is normal and the metaphysis appears flared.

Rickets Slide I,27 shows the radiographic and histologic features of rickets. In rickets, a calcifiable matrix is formed, but it does not calcify. The primary spongiosum is not formed and the osteoid in the metaphysis is not mineralized. The hypertrophic zone is greatly widened and tongues of cartilage extend into the metaphysis. Vascular invasion is thwarted, and the vascular loops are turned aside, as depicted in Slide I,28. The bone that does form is thin and sparse. The radiographic findings in rickets include no zone of provisional calcification, increased separation between the epiphysis and the diaphysis, and flaring of the metaphysis.

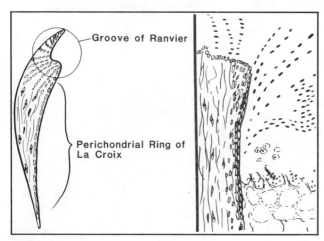

Slide I,25

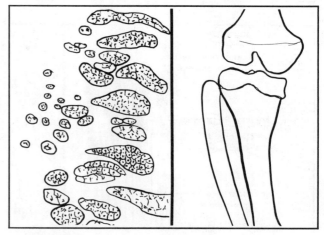

Slide I,26

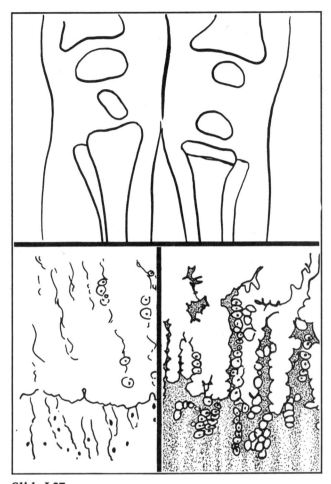

Slide I,27

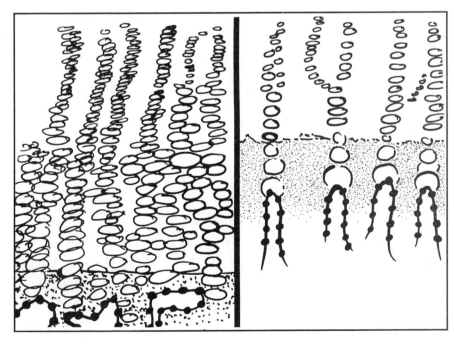

Slide I,28

Osteogenesis imperfecta Osteogenesis imperfecta is a systemic, connective tissue disorder, the manifestations of which are shown radiographically and histologically in Slide I,29. Osteogenesis imperfecta is a primary disease of osteoblasts. Much of the collagen elaborated by the cells never matures beyond the reticulum stage. The cartilage of the growth plate appears normal, but the secondary spongiosum is defective because very little new bone is deposited on the calcified cartilage bars. The bony trabeculae formed are thin and fragile. Radiographic examination shows thin cortices, poor trabeculation in the metaphysis, and often fractures in various stages of healing.

Osteopetrosis The histologic and radiographic appearance of osteopetrosis is seen in Slide I,30. Osteopetrosis (marble bone disease or Albers-Schönberg disease) is a failure of the osteoclast to resorb bone. The growth plate is normal down to the primary spongiosum. The calcified cartilage bars in this layer are not absorbed or removed. Primitive osseous tissue is laid down on the cartilage remnants, never converting to mature lamellar bone. Such bar remnants are found throughout the entire length of bone, including the midshaft. As bone growth proceeds, no true medullary cavity is formed. Radiographic examination characteristically shows uniform opacity of the severely involved bones, with no discernible internal architecture. The lack of external remodeling prevents normal funnelization of the metaphysis.

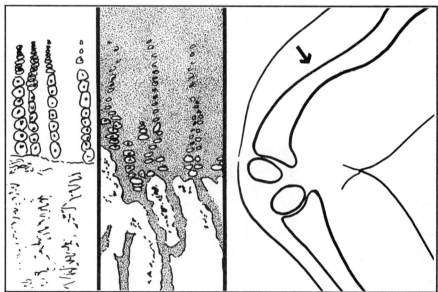

Slide I,29

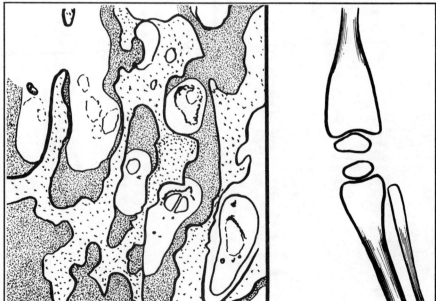

Slide I,30

Form and Function of Articular Cartilage

Morphology

Articular cartilage is avascular and alymphatic. Hence, nutrients are diffused through the matrix. Diffusion is highly dependent on joint motion and compression loads. Articular cartilage is also aneural, so injuries to the cartilage are not directly detected by the organism.

In the growing child, the cartilage at the ends of long bones performs two functions. The superficial portion acts as a load bearing articular surface in much the same fashion as adult cartilage. The deeper zone is the growth plate of the epiphysis. The epiphyseal growth plate portion functions to cause the lengthening of the bone by endochondral bone formation and to increase the width of the joint surface by both appositional chondrogenesis and by proliferation of the chondrocytes within the matrix of the growth plate. At puberty, the growth plate is obliterated, and only the articular cartilage remains to cover the end of the bone.

Adult articular cartilage varies in thickness from 2 to 4 mm. Across any articular surface the thickness also varies and is greater at the periphery of concave surfaces (glenoid) and near the center of convex joint surfaces (patellar). Slide I,31 is a histologic composite showing the zones of adult articular cartilage. The superficial tangential zone (STZ) consists of collagen fibers randomly woven but horizontally oriented. This weave appears very coarse when viewed by the scanning electron microscope, and the site of the spaces, or pores between the fibers is critical to the lubrication of the joint. The collagen arches downward (central slide) through the transitional zone or upper middle zone and into the zone of calcified cartilage below. As the orientation of the collagen becomes more vertical, so does the apparent orientation of the chondrocyte. Also, the chondrocytes in the superficial zone appear flattened, whereas in the deeper zones they are rounder. The cells of adult articular cartilage do not appear to replicate under normal circumstances, which does not mean the cells are dormant. Chondrocytes continue to demonstrate synthetic activity as shown by Na_2 $^{35}SO_4$ radioisotope studies.

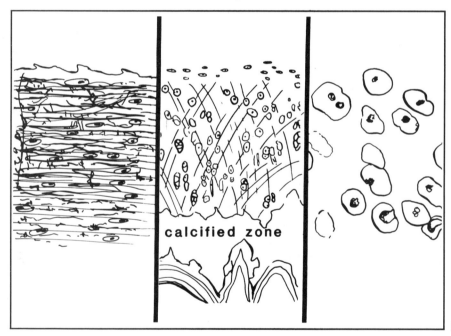

calcified zone

Slide I,31

The deepest zone of adult articular cartilage is calcified. The mineral density is greatest at the interface of the calcified zone with the supporting subchondral cortex and least at the surface. This gradient serves to protect the collagen fibers from shear forces. The zone of calcified cartilage shown histologically and diagrammatically in I,32 is metabolically active, and increases with age, reducing the relative thickness of the articular cartilage.

Constituents of Cartilage

It is possible to describe the constituents of cartilage (water, collagen, proteoglycans, glycoproteins, cells), but it should be clear that these components are non-uniformly distributed throughout articular cartilage. The non-uniform distribution makes possible both the unique weight-bearing capabilities and the lubrication of synovial joints. Anatomically, these unique structural properties of cartilage orient the functional behavior of the tissue.

Each of the constituents of cartilage contributes something to its function. The chondrocytes replenish degraded proteoglycans and collagen. Proteoglycans withstand compressive loads and swell again when the load is released, as shown in Slide I,33. Collagen withstands tensile stresses, and although age detracts from the strength, collagen together with proteoglycans can protect cartilage from shear for many years.

Slide I,34 is a diagram of a proteoglycan aggregate. Proteoglycans are the major organic macromolecules of the cartilage gel matrix. Proteoglycans consist of glycosaminoglycan side chains attached to a central protein core. The glycosaminoglycan side chains are keratan sulfate, chondroitin-4 sulfate, and chondroitin-6 sulfate. The protein core of the subunit is in turn attached to a hyaluronic acid core via a special "link" protein. The negatively charged side chains of this molecule shown at the bottom of Slide I,34 repel each other. The charged side chains attract water, resulting in a large solute domain for the subunit.

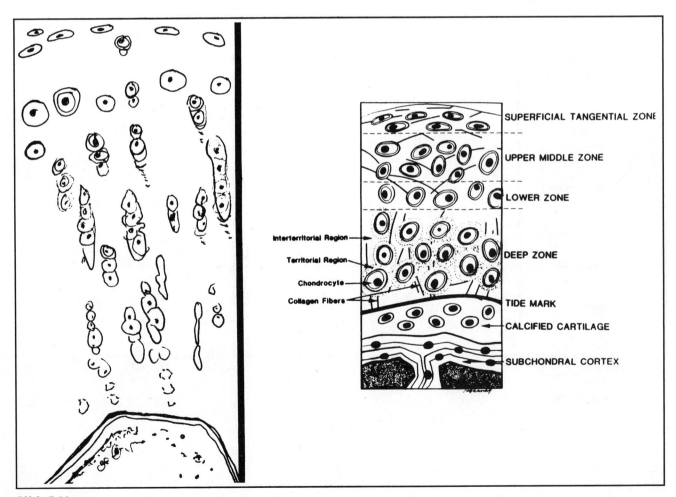

Slide I,32

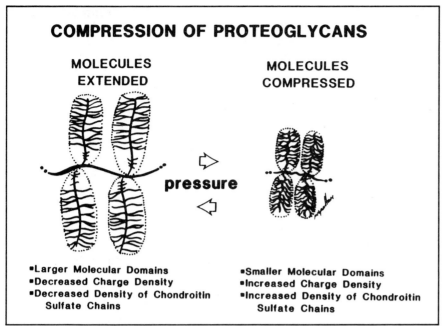

COMPRESSION OF PROTEOGLYCANS

MOLECULES EXTENDED

MOLECULES COMPRESSED

pressure

- Larger Molecular Domains
- Decreased Charge Density
- Decreased Density of Chondroitin Sulfate Chains

- Smaller Molecular Domains
- Increased Charge Density
- Increased Density of Chondroitin Sulfate Chains

Slide I,33

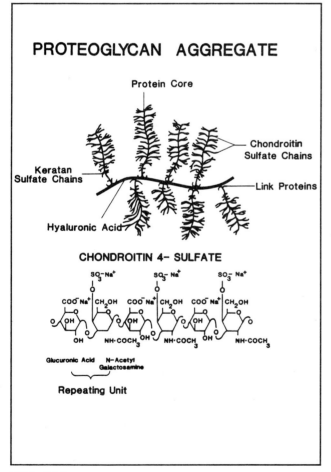

PROTEOGLYCAN AGGREGATE

Protein Core

Chondroitin Sulfate Chains

Keratan Sulfate Chains

Link Proteins

Hyaluronic Acid

CHONDROITIN 4- SULFATE

Glucuronic Acid   N–Acetyl Galactosamine

Repeating Unit

Slide I,34

The serpentine proteoglycan molecule and its subunits are shown diagrammatically in Slide I,35. The proteoglycan appears not to bind directly to collagen, but to intertwine among the collagen fibers. The collagen fiber network, as shown in Slide I,36 is sufficiently dense to constrain and contain the proteoglycan aggregates, trapping the proteoglycans within the articular cartilage envelope. The proteoglycans, attempting to gain the solute domain, apply tensile forces to the collagen fibers, as illustrated in Slide I,37. The swelling of the proteoglycans against the surrounding collagen helps to maintain the spatial form of articular cartilage. The distention or expansion of cartilage by the proteoglycans is a measurable force called the swelling pressure.

If the surface of cartilage is pierced multiply, each joint surface in the body can be shown to have a specific and repeatable split line pattern. Slide I,38 illustrates such a pattern in the distal femoral condyle. This non-uniform orientation of cartilage components demonstrates properties that vary depending on the direction and speed of the applied forces.

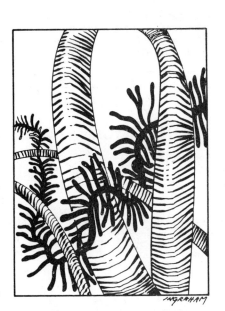

Slide I,35

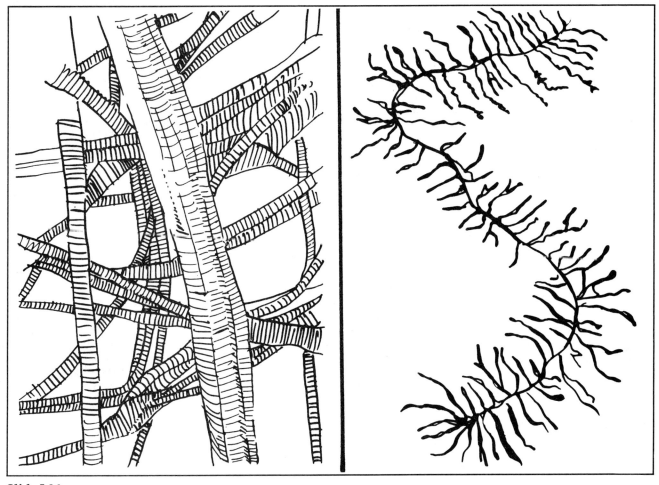

Slide I,36

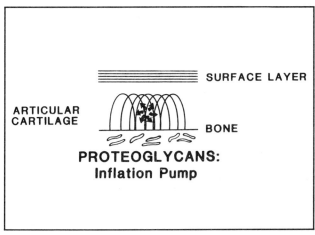

ARTICULAR
CARTILAGE

SURFACE LAYER

BONE

PROTEOGLYCANS:
Inflation Pump

Slide I,37

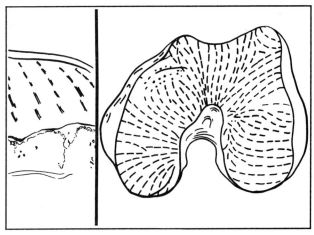

Slide I,38

Meniscus

Menisci are disc-shaped, fibrocartilaginous structures occurring in the acromioclavicular and sternoclavicular, glenohumeral, hip, and knee joints. Meniscal structures broaden the contact region of synovial joints and provide a wider cross-sectional area upon which to support loads.

Structure and Composition

Menisci are firm semi-lunar structures the triangular shape of which is derived embryologically from the mesenchyme separating the rounded margins of articular cartilage at the edges of joints. As such, they fully occupy the potential space between the joint surfaces.

Slide I,39 depicts the collagen fiber arrangement in the menisci. The collagen is predominately type I and is similar to that found in bone, in contrast to type II collagen found in articular cartilage. Type III is also found, as are small quantities of V and II-like collagen. In the most superficial layer, the fibers are predominately radially oriented. Beneath the radial fibers are large bundles of collagen circumferentially arranged, as shown in Slide I,40. Even in this deeper zone, the huge bundles appear to be interlaced with random branch fibers that may serve to link the main fiber bundles, as shown in Slide I,41. Obviously, fiber bundles this thick can resist circumferential, or "hoop" stresses. Menisci can be shown to have radially oriented split lines. Weight loading of the meniscus by the femoral condyle causes radial displacement resisted by the radially oriented collagen fibers. Failure of these fibers can result in a meniscus tear.

Menisci are 70% water. Although the central portion of the triangular meniscus has a high concentration of proteoglycans, they constitute only 2.5% of the solid matrix, one-tenth the amount found in articular cartilage.

Nutrition

The nutrition of menisci is only partly due to diffusion and weight bearing. Diffusion of nutrients is limited to a depth of one millimeter from the surface. Menisci retain about 20% of their embryonic mesenchymal blood supply, as shown by India-ink injection in Slide I,42. Vascularization is present in the outer 20% to 30% of the meniscus. Knowledge of this vascular arborization permits repair of selected peripheral meniscus tears. Cells of the menisci are limited to those areas supplied by blood vessels or diffusion.

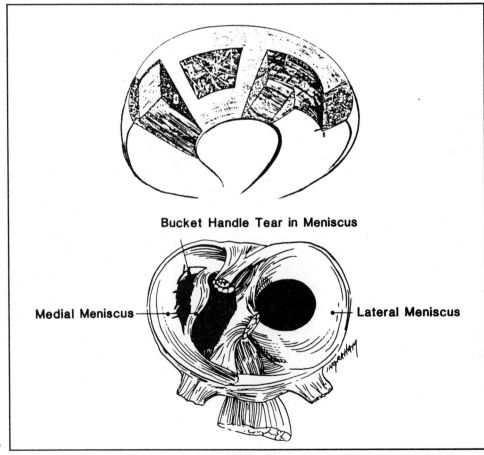

Bucket Handle Tear in Meniscus

Medial Meniscus —   Lateral Meniscus

Slide I,39

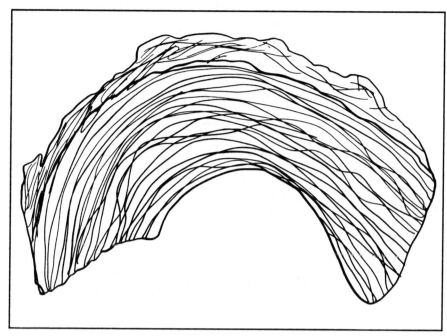

Slide I,40

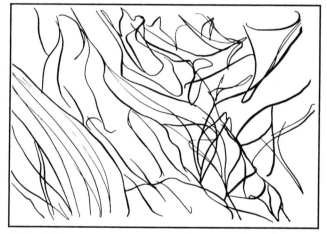

Slide I,41

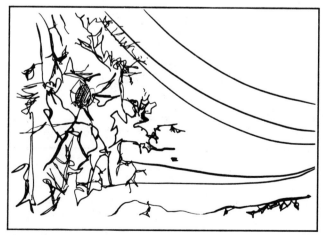

Slide I,42

Muscle

Morphologically, muscles can be classified into a variety of types based on their general form and fascicular architecture. In general, the closer the fibers come to a longitudinal orientation the greater the range of motion. The more they deviate from a longitudinal array, e.g., multipennate, the stronger the muscle. Although individual muscle fibers can contract approximately one half of their resting length, only perfectly longitudinally arranged muscles can approximate this contraction.

Slide I,43 illustrates the wide variety of fiber orientations including parallel, fusiform, unipennate, bipennate, triangular, and spiral. In addition, some of the fibers between their attachments may be spiraled or twisted. Slide I,44 depicts the breakdown of a muscle from the gross muscle level to the contractile protein (myofilament) level.

Slide I,45 is a hematoxylin and eosin stain of longitudinally cut muscle revealing the multinucleated striated appearance of skeletal muscle fibers. The striations result from the organization of the contractile proteins.

As seen in cross section on Slide I,46, the connective tissue components, epimysium, perimysium, and endomysium are illustrated, along with the capillary bed. Cross sections such as this one provide an accurate way to measure muscle fiber size (atrophy or hypertrohy) to determine if the nuclei are in their normal peripheral locations. With special stains, muscle fiber types can be identified.

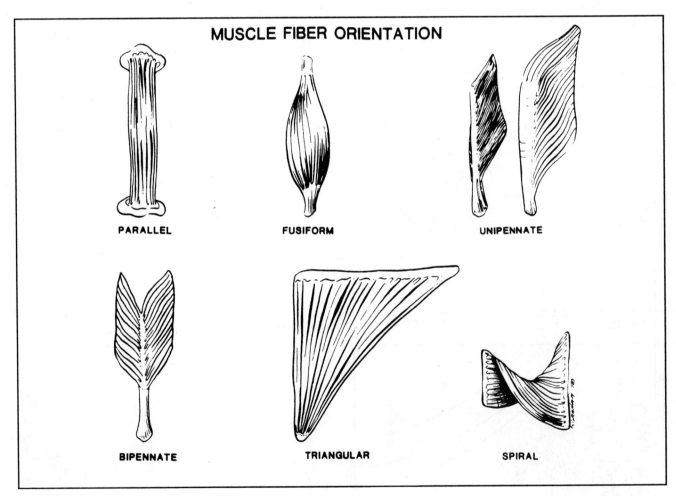

MUSCLE FIBER ORIENTATION

PARALLEL   FUSIFORM   UNIPENNATE

BIPENNATE   TRIANGULAR   SPIRAL

Slide I,43

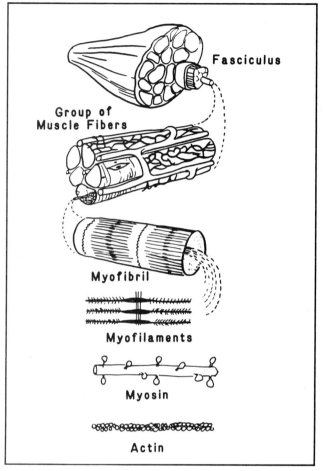

Slide I,44

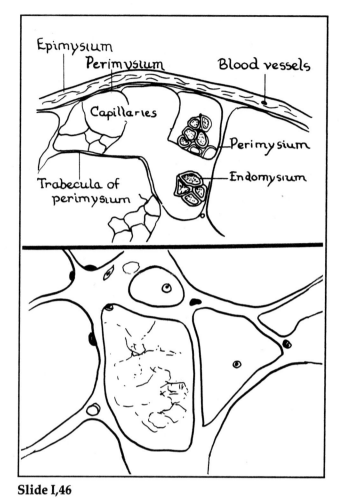

Slide I,46

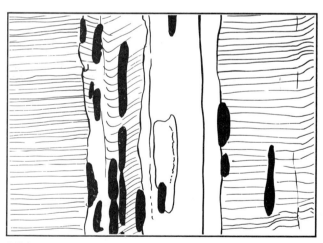

Slide I,45

Muscle fibers have been classified by a wide variety of schemes, but two such schemes tend to persist. These are types I and II; slow twitch oxidative (SO), and fast twitch glycolytic (FG), or fast twitch oxidative-glycolytic (FOG). In relating the two schemes, type I refers to the slow twitch fibers that contain high oxidative enzyme content, (SO), whereas type II fibers imply fast twitch fibers with high ATP-ase content and low oxidative enzyme content (FG).

Typical staining patterns to delineate muscle fiber types are illustrated in Slide I,47. Left, SDH reaction—dark fibers = SO or type I; light fibers = FG or type II fibers. Right, ATP-ase reaction—dark fibers = FG or type II; light fibers = SO or type I. SO fibers have high oxidative enzyme levels, low myosin ATP-ase and glycogen levels, slow contraction-relaxation curves, and are very resistant to fatigue. FG fibers have high myosin ATP-ase and glycogen levels, fast contraction-relaxation curves, and fatigue quickly. FOG fibers have high levels of myosin ATP-ase, oxidation enzymes and glycogen, fairly rapid contraction-relaxation curves, and fatigue more slowly than FG fibers.

The types I and II scheme generally refers to the SO and FG fibers, respectively. FOG fibers are not as prevalent and cannot be identified unless both oxidative and ATP-ase staining are done, since FOG fibers have high oxidative enzyme content, which would make them type I fibers, but they also have high ATP-ase reactions, which would classify them as type II fibers.

Other properties associated with the different fiber types are outlined in Slides I,48, I,49, and I,50.

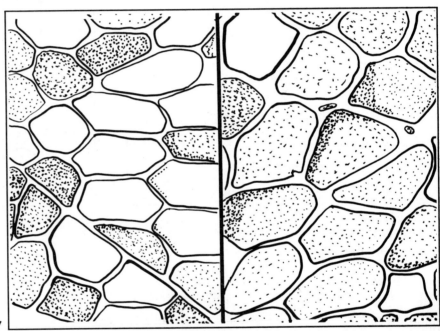

Slide I,47

FIBER TYPE

II	II	I
–FAST-TWITCH	FAST-TWITCH	SLOW-TWITCH
– WHITE	RED	INTERMED.
– FAST-TWITCH	FAST-TWITCH	SLOW-TWITCH
GLYCOLYTIC	OXIDATIVE	OXIDATIVE
	GLYCOLYTIC	

Slide I,48

ENZYMATIC PROPERTIES

–OXIDATIVE ENZYME ACTIVITES	LOW	HIGH	INT.–HIGH
–GLYCOLYTIC ACTIVITIES	HIGH	INT.–LOW	LOW–VARIABLE
–MYOFIBRILLAR ATPASE	HIGH	HIGH	LOW
–GLYCOGEN CONTENT	INT.	HIGH	LOW

Slide I,49

PHYSICAL PROPERTIES

–FIBER DIAMETER	LARGE	SMALL	INTER.
–MYOGLOBIN	LOW	HIGH	HIGH
–VELOCITY OF CONTRACTION	FAST	FAST	SLOW
–FATIGABILITY	SUSCEPTIBLE	LESS SUSCEPTIBLE	CONTRACTS INDEFINITE
–COLOR (Macroscopic)	WHITE	RED	RED

Slide I,50

Slide I,51 illustrates the ultrastructure of myofibrils consisting of the longitudinally arranged sarcomere. Each sarcomere runs from Z-band to Z-band and is divided into I-bands and A-bands. The Z-bands consist of the protein alpha actinin; the I-bands consist of actin and tropomyosin, and troponin; and the A-bands consist of the actin-tropomyosin-troponin couples and myosin. In the center of the A-band is the H-zone representing that part of the A-band consisting only of myosin. In the contracted state, the H-zone is a darker line (M-line) due to cross-bridge attachments between myosin molecules.

Between adjacent myofibrils, elements of the conducting system (sarcoplasmic reticulum) and cytoplasmic organelles can be identified. At the A-I band junction in mammals, T-tubules project inward from the sarcolemma surrounding each myofibril. As depolarization of the sarcolemma occurs, it passes inward at each T-tube and is then transferred out across the sarcoplasmic reticulum (SR) between the T-tubules, releasing stored calcium ions from the SR. At relaxation, the calcium is taken back up by the SR. The junction between the T-tubules and the SR constitutes a *triad*. Scattered among the tubular system are mitochondria, ribosomes, and glycogen.

Skeletal muscle is innervated by a wide variety of neurons. Motor neurons supplying the motor end plates belong to the A-alpha class. A-gamma neurons supply motor endings to the intrafusal muscle fibers comprising muscle spindles. A-beta neurons are rare in humans but common in amphibians. They branch to send motor endings to both skeletal muscle fibers (extrafusal fibers) and muscle spindles (intrafusal fibers [IF]). Classes B and C efferent neurons are associated with the autonomic nervous system (ANS). Sensory neurons are classified as I, II, III and IV. Class I is further subdivided into I-a

(primary sensory endings to muscle spindles) and I-b (golgi-tendon organs [GTO]). Class II endings are secondary endings to muscle spindles and Class III and IV neurons are associated with pain, touch, and pressure. Slide I,52 lists some of the characteristics of the different nerve fibers.

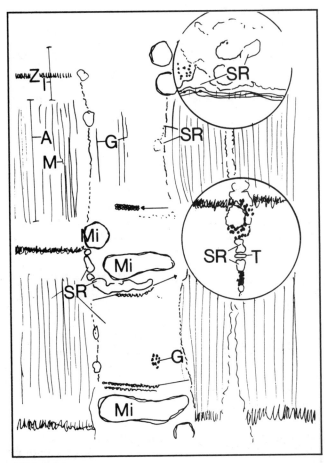

Slide I,51

The distribution of these neurons in skeletal muscle is illustrated diagrammatically in Slide I,53. In terms of proportion, cat soleus studies have indicated that the muscle contains approximately 25,000 muscle fibers, and the tibial nerve to the soleus consists of 390 neurons. Of these, 150 are A-alpha supplying the extrafusal motor end plates, and 240 neurons are either I-a, II or A-gamma fibers for sensory control mechanisms. Therefore, 60% of the neurons are associated with sensory receptor mechanisms, whereas 40% are involved with direct motor innervation. The number of muscle fibers supplied by one A-alpha neuron constitutes a motor unit. All muscle fibers of a single motor unit will be the same fiber type, since it is the frequency of impulses coming through the motor axon that determines fiber type.

MOTOR

GROUP	DIAMETER	VELOCITY	TERMINATION
A α	12–20	60–100	• MUSCLE FIBERS
β	6–12	30–70	• AXONS TO SPINDLE IF's
γ	2 8	15–30	• SPINDLE IF's
δ	2–6	12–30	• (BLOOD VESSELS ?)
B	1–3	3–15	• ANS PREGANGLIONIC
C	.5–1	.5–2	• ANS POSTGANGLIONIC

SENSORY

GROUP	DIAMETER	VELOCITY	ORIGIN (Receptors)
Ia Ib	12–22	70–120	• SPINDLE, GTO, JOINT
II	6–12	30–70	• SPINDLE, SKIN, JOINT
III	2–6	12–30	• PAIN
IV	.5–1	.5–2	• PAIN

Slide I,52

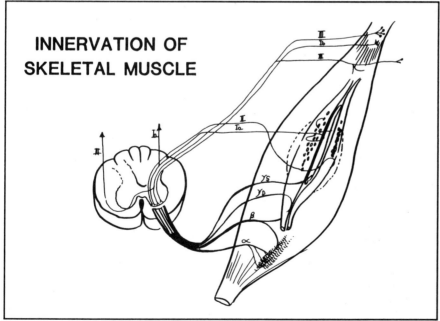

INNERVATION OF SKELETAL MUSCLE

Slide I,53

A typical motor unit consisting of one A-alpha axon branching to supply four motor endplates on four muscle fibers is illustrated in Slide I,54. This motor unit is, therefore, one axon and four muscle fibers. Motor units may exist in a 1:1 ratio with muscle fibers or 1:>100 depending on the muscle involved. The details of the motor end plate are seen by electron microscopy in Slide I,55 [SC-Schwann cell, Gu=gutter, JF=junctional folds, M=mitochondria, NE=nerve ending, BM=basement membrane, CT=connective tissue (endomysium), *=myofibrils].

A final structure typical of all skeletal muscle is the satellite cell, as seen in Slide I,56. These cells are nearly impossible to identify by light microscopy since they are located peripherally and consist of a single nucleus with scanty cytoplasm. Therefore, they appear as normal muscle nuclei. By electron microscopy the separation of cell membranes between the muscle fiber and the satellite cell can be seen. These cells are important in the process of muscle regeneration as a source of new muscle fiber nuclei.

The Blix length-tension curve is shown in Slide I,57. The maximum force a muscle can develop varies with its initial length. The maximum contractile force produced by a muscle is at its resting length.

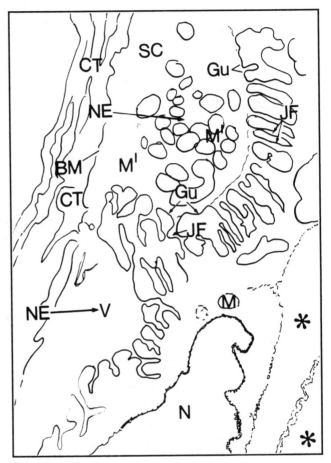

Slide I,55

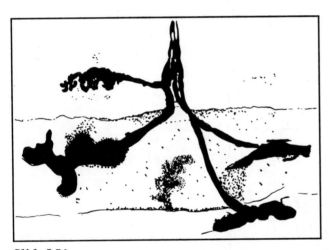

Slide I,54

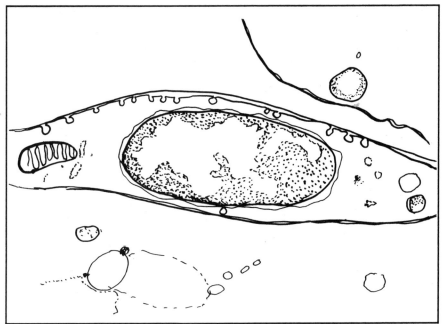

Slide I,56

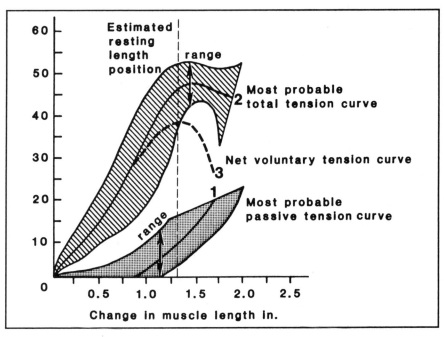

Slide I,57

Tendon

Tendons are dense, regularly arranged collagenous structures connecting muscles to bone. Tendons must resist large longitudinal tensile stresses.

As illustrated in Slide I,58, the collagen fibers insert directly into bone. However, if relatively soft collagen fibers insert into relatively rigid bones, the repeated bending and stretching of tendons near bones would cause failure. To dissipate the stresses, tendons have a transitional calcified zone, which has an increasing density of calcium as the tendon nears its bony insertion.

When transferring a tendon, a "shingle" of cortical bone has traditionally been a technique used to unite collagen to bone and to provide an interface for transmission of forces from the soft tendon to the hard bone. Slide I,59 shows that the principal cell in tendon is the fibroblast. The fibroblast lies between collagen bundles. The lateral limits of the cell are not discernible because the cell processes extend out between the collagen bundles. Fibroblasts elaborate the matrix of tendons, collagen and glycoproteins. The glycoproteins are not as abundant as in articular cartilage.

The principal component of tendon is type I collagen. Slide I,60 demonstrates the in-register arrangement of the aggregated collagen fibers, which on the ultrastructural level creates a stable biologic unit of very great strength. Slide I,61 illustrates the composition of a typical tendon.

Tendons that are not enclosed within a sheath are surrounded by loose areolar connective tissue called the paratenon. The paratenon surrounds tendons that move in a straight line and consists of elastic fibers and somewhat coiled blood vessels that can stretch out during elongation of the tendon.

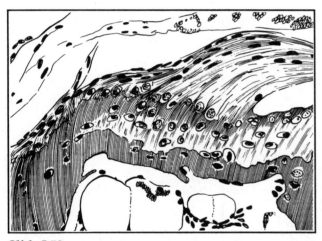

Slide I,58

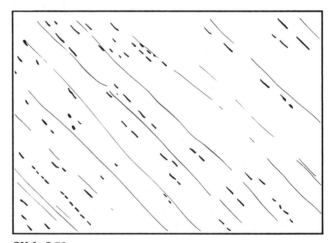

Slide I,59

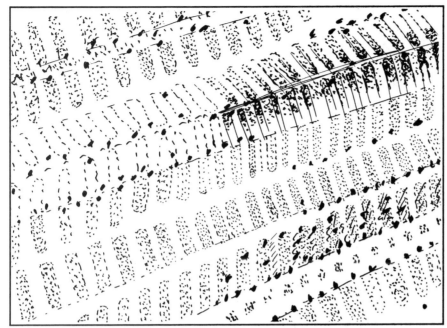

Slide I,60

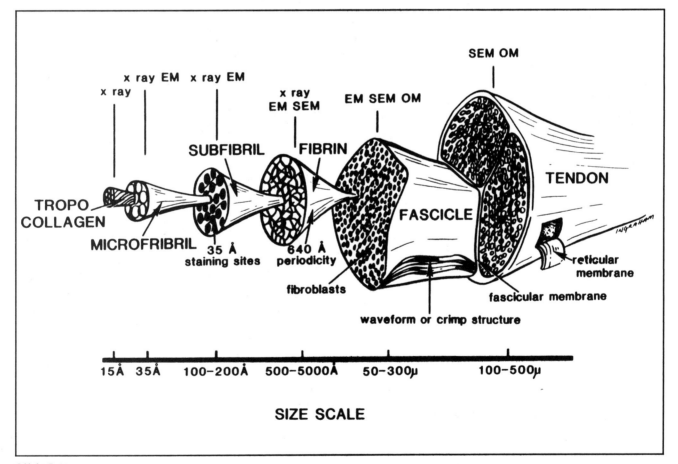

Slide I,61

Tendons which bend sharply around corners, such as the flexor tendons of the hand, or the toe flexors, are suspended by pulleys and are enclosed by a sheath to prevent bowstringing of the tendon. A bifoliate mesotenon originates opposite the site of friction, and joins the epitenon to form a sheath. Slide I,62 shows this arrangement in a tendon undergoing repair. The gliding of the tendon is assisted by synovial fluid, extruded from the parietal and the visceral synovial membranes of the epitenon.

Tendons receive their blood supply from the perimysium, periosteal attachments, and surrounding tissue. The blood supply from surrounding soft tissues reaches the tendon through the paratenon, mesotenon or the vincula, as shown in Slide I,63. A distinction has been made between so-called vascular and avascular tendons. "Vascular" tendons are surrounded by a paratenon and receive vessels all along their borders. The vessels then arborize within the tendon as shown in Slide I,64. "Avascular" tendons are contained within tendon sheaths and the mesotenons are reduced to the vascularized conduits called vincula.

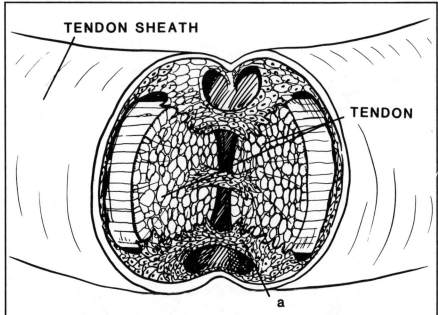

Slide I,62

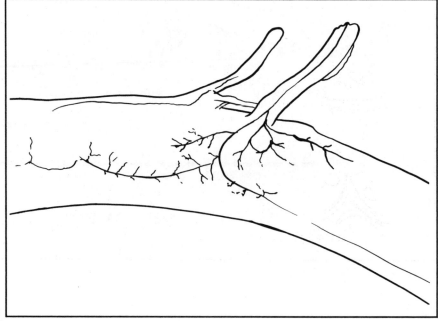

Slide I,63

Nerve

Slide I,65 illustrates the connective tissue arrangement of a peripheral nerve. (Ep=epineurium, Pe=perineurium, En=endoneurium, Fa=fascicle, NF=individual neurons, BV=blood vessels.) The peripheral nerve consists of bundles of axons enclosed within connective tissue sheaths, the epineurium. The perineurium divides the axon into bundles of fascicles and the endoneurium surrounds individual axons. These connective tissue components are important in protecting individual axons and groups of axons from injury. Most (mixed) peripheral nerves consist of all the types of neurons described in the innervation of skeletal muscle.

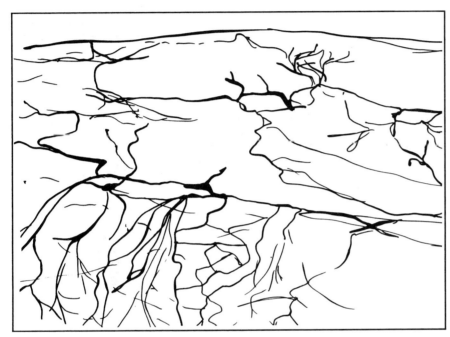

Slide I,64

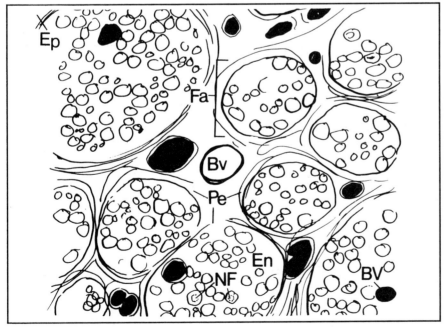

Slide I,65

Most neurons are myelinated, as shown in Slide I,66. Myelination means that Schwann cell cytoplasm wraps around the axon many times, resulting in close apposition of the inner and outer layers of the Schwann cell membrane, illustrated in Slide I,66 and in higher magnification at the upper left corner of the slide. Nonmyelinated neurons actually are encased only by a single layer of Schwann cell cytoplasm (neurolemma). The gaps between Schwann cells constitute the nodes of Ranvier.

Depolarization occurs in the region of the nodes. A typical node is illustrated in Slide I,67. [SC=Schwann cell; CT=connective tissue (endoneurium); My=myelin; Nf=neurofilaments; M=mitochondria; BM=basement membrane; ER=endoplasmic reticulum; X=folds of Schwann cell cytoplasm at the node; Pr=processes of Schwann cell cytoplasm covering the node in a monolayer.]

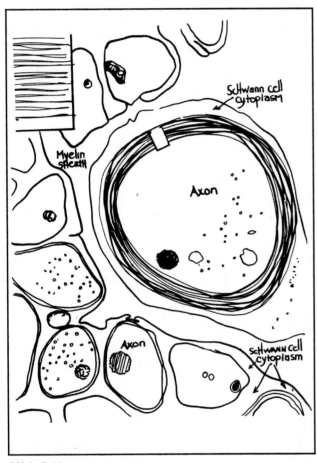

Slide I,66

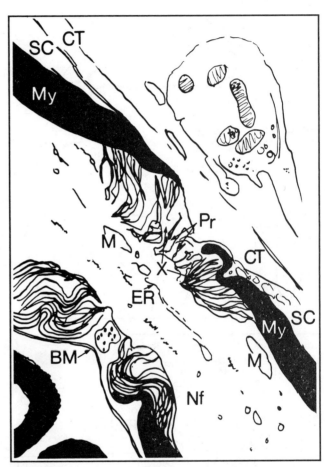

Slide I,67

Selected Bibliography

Bone

Skeletal Research: An Experimental Approach, Simmons D, Kumin A (eds): New York, Academic Press, 1979.

Thyberg J: Electron microscopic studies of the initial phases of calcification in guinea pig epiphyseal cartilage. J Ultrastruct Res 1974; 46:206-218.

Thyberg J: Electron microscopic and cytochemical studies of the guinea pig metaphysis with special reference to the lysosomal system of different cell types. Cell Tiss Res 1975; 156:273-279.

Thyberg J: Electron microscopic studies on the uptake of exogenous marker particles by different cell types in the guinea pig metaphysis. Cell Tiss Res 1975; 156: 301-315.

Tonna E: Electron microscopy of aging skeletal cells III. Periosteum Lab Invest 1974; 31:609-632.

Mineralization

Bosky AL: Current concepts of the biochemistry and physiology of calcification. Clin Orthop 1981; 157: 165-196.

Wuthier RE: A review of the primary mechanism of endochondral calcification with special emphasis on the role of the cells, mitochondria, and matrix vesicles. Clin Orthop 1982; 169:219-242.

Articular Cartilage

Armstrong CG, Mow VC: Variations in the intrinsic mechanical properties of human articular cartilage with age, degeneration, and water content. J Bone Joint Surg 1982; 64A:88-94.

Benninghoff A: Form und bau der gelenkenknorpel in ihren beziehungen zur funktion. Zweiter Teil: Zeitschrift fur Zellforschung und mikorskopische Anatomie 1925; 2:783.

Bullough PG, Goodfellow J: The significance of the fine structure of articular cartilage. J Bone Joint Surg 1968; 50-B:852.

Dmitrovsky E, Lane LB, Bullough PG: The characterization of the tidemark in human articular cartilage. Metab Bone Dis and Rel Res 1978; 1:115.

Adult Articular Cartilage, Freeman MAR (ed): London, Pittman, 1979

Lane LB, Villacin A, Bullough PG: The vascularity and remodeling of subchondral bone and calcified cartilage in adult human femoral and humeral heads: an age and stress-related phenomenon. J Bone Joint Surg 1977; 59-B:272.

Mankin HJ: Mitosis in articular cartilage of immature rabbits: a histologic, stathmokinetic (colchicinic) and autoradiograph study. Clin Orthop 1964; 34:170-183.

Mankin HJ, Dorfman H, Lippiello L, et al: Biochemical and metabolic abnormalities in articular cartilage from osteo-arthritc human hips. Correlation of morphology and biochemical and metabolic data. J Bone Joint Surg 1971; 53A:523-537.

Mankin HJ, Lippiello L: The turnover of adult rabbit articular cartilage. J Bone Joint Surg 1969; 51A: 1591-1600.

Maroudas A: Cartilage turnover. Ann Rheum Dis 1975; 34(Suppl2):5-57.

Mow VC, Schoonbeck JM: Contribution of Donnan osmotic pressure towards the biphasic compressive modulus of articular cartilage. Trans Orthop Res Soc 1984; 9:262.

Muir H: Proteoglycans as organizers of the intercellular matrix. Biochem Soc Trans 1983; 11:613-622.

Muir IHM: The chemistry of the ground substance of joint cartilage, in L Sokoloff (ed): The Joints and Synovial Fluid, Vol II, New York, Academic Press, 1980, pp 27-94.

Myers ER: Kinetic and equilibrium swelling studies of connective tissues. Doctoral Thesis, Rensselaer Polytechnic Institute, Troy NY, 1984.

Ogaton A: On the growth and maintenance of the articular ends of adult bones. J Anat and Physiol 1878; XII:503.

Rosenberg LC: Proteoglycans, in Owen R, Goodfellow JW, Bullough PG (eds): The Scientific Foundations of Orthopaedics and Traumatology, Philadelphia and Toronto, WB Saunders, 1980, pp 36-42.

Stockwell RA, Meachim G: The chondrocytes, in Freeman MAR (ed):Adult Articular Cartilage. London, Pittman, 1979, p 69.

Sapolsky AI, Howell DS, Woessner JF: Neutral proteases and cathepsin-D in human articular cartilage. J Clin Invest 1974; 53:1044-1053.

Venn MF: Variation of chemical composition with age in human femoral head cartilage. Ann Rheum Dis 1978; 37:168-174.

Wirth CR, Augello FA, Mow VC, et al: Variation of tensile properties of human patellar cartilage with age and indices. Orth Res Soc Trans 1980; 5:38.

Menisci

Adams ME, Muir H: The glycosaminoglycans of canine menisci. Biochem J 1981; 197:385-389.

Ahmed AM, Burke DL: In-vivo measurement of static pressure distribution in synovial joints, part I. Tibial surface of the knee. J Biomech Eng 1983; 105:216-225.

Aroncsky SP, Marshall JL, Joseph A, et al: Meniscal nutrition — an experimental study in the dog. Trans Orthop Res Soc 1980; 5:127.

Aronczky SP, Warren RF: Microvasculature of the human meniscus. Am J Sports Med 1982; 10:90-95.

Bullough PG, Munuera L, Murphy J, et al: The strength of the meniscus of the knee as it relates to their fine structure. J Bone Joint Surg 1970; 52-B:564-570.

Eyre DR, Wu JJ: Collagen of fibrocartilage: a distinctive molecular phenotype in bovine meniscus. FEBS Letters 1983; 158:265-270.

Fairbanks TJ: Knee joint changes after meniscectomy. J Bone Joint Surg 1936; 18:333-342.

Livingston R, Wirth CR: Meniscal vasculature and repair. Contemporary Orthopaedics 1984; 8:39-43.

McNichol D, Roughly PJ: The presence of a cartilage-like proteoglycan from the human meniscus. Trans Orthop Res Soc 1980; 5:150.

Mow VC, Keui S, Lai WM, et al: Biphasic creep and stress relaxation of articular cartilage in compression: theory and experiments. J Biochem Eng 1980; 102:73-84.

Roughly PJ, McNichol D, Santer V, et al: The presence of cartilage-like proteoglycan in the adult human meniscus. Biochem J 1981; 197:77-83.

Scapinelli R: Studies on the vasculature of the human knee. Acta Anat Basel 1968; 70:305-331.

Wirth CR: Meniscus Repair. Clin Orthop 1981; 157: 153-160.

Whipple R, Mow VC, Wirth CR: Anisotrophic and zonal variations in the tensile properties of the meniscus. Trans Ortho Res Soc 1985; 10:367.

Muscle and Nerve

Engle WK: Selective and nonselective susceptibility of muscle fiber types. A new approach to human neuromuscular diseases. Ann Neurology 1970; 22:97-117.

Matthews PBC: Muscle spindles and their motor control. Physiol Rev 1964; 44:219-288.

Ovalle WK, Jr: Motor nerve terminals on rat intrafusal muscle fibers, a correlated light and electron microscopic study. J Anat 1972; 111:239-252.

Porter KR, Bonneville MA: Fine Structure of Cells and Tissues. Philadelphia, Lea and Febiger, 1968.

Rhodin JAG: An Atlas of Histology. New York, Oxford Univ Press, 1975.

Tomanek RJ, Lund DD: Degeneration of different types of skeletal muscle fibers II. Immobilization. J Anat 1974; 118:531-541.

Tendon

Cooper RR, Misol S: Tendon and ligament insertion. J Bone Joint Surg 1970; 52-A:1-19.

Lundborg G, Myrhage R: The vascularization and structure of the human digital tendon sheath as related to flexor tendon function. Scand J Plastic Surg 1977; 11: 195-203.

Chapter II

Disorders of Bone

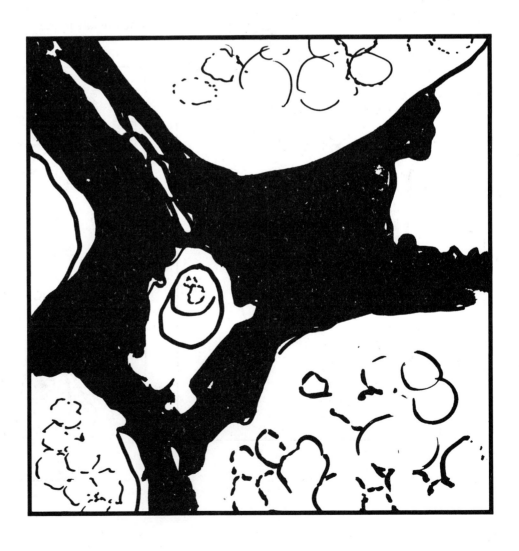

Basic scientific investigation during the past 25 years has enhanced the understanding of bone remodeling, bone metabolism and homeostasis, metabolic bone disorders, bone repair, bone grafting, and genetically induced disorders of bone. This chapter presents a basic discussion of these topics with the intention of providing the orthopaedist with a sound scientific basis for clinical management and decision making.

Bone Remodeling

External Modeling And Remodeling

Slide II,1 shows the head and neck of the femur, illustrating quite well the general principle that the external form and shape of a bone as an organ, and the internal organization of bone as a tissue are both very well adapted to the forces placed upon them. The upper figure shows the lines of force throughout the proximal femur, while the lower figure demonstrates the bony trabeculae aligned along the lines of stress.

The ability of bone to remodel itself both externally and internally is vitally important to its mechanical functions. The amount of bone mass, its organization and distribution, and the orientation of the trabeculae are all sensitive to the amount and kind of stress applied to bone. Hypertrophy of bone, atrophy of bone, and external remodeling in fracture repair are common examples of bone's response to loading known as Wolff's law.

Remodeling of bone takes place throughout the life of the individual. Slide II,2 illustrates the effects of age on the metacarpal cortex (top) and femoral diaphysis (bottom). With age, the endosteal (inner) diameter and the periosteal (outer) diameter of long bones gradually increase in men and women. In women at menopause, the endosteal diameter increases more rapidly than the periosteal diameter, leading to an appreciable net decrease in cortical thickness. The same phenomenon occurs in men but at a slower rate.

A 10% increase in the periosteal diameter places the cortex farther from the central axis of the bone and compensates in terms of bending forces for a 30% loss of bone mass. Torque loads are not comparably protected, however. Consequently, there is an increased fracture rate in the elderly consistent with the net cortical bone loss.

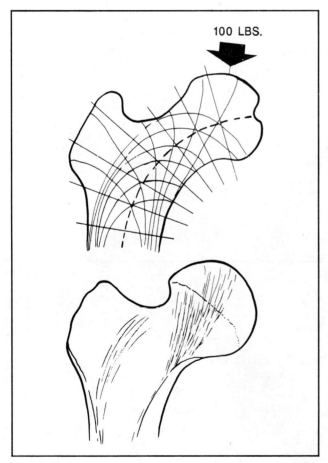

Slide II,1

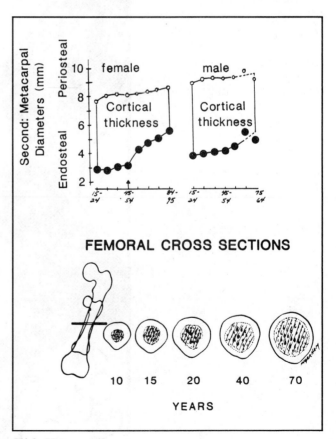

Slide II,2

Internal Cortical and Trabecular Remodeling

Cortical bone constitutes approximately 80% of the skeletal mass and trabecular bone approximately 20%. Bone surfaces may be undergoing formation, resorption, or they may be inactive. These proceses occur in both cortical and trabecular bone throughout life. Bone remodeling is a surface phenomenon and occurs on periosteal, endosteal, haversian canal, and trabecular surfaces. The rate of cortical bone remodeling may be as high as 50% per year in the midshaft of the femur during the first two years of life, but eventually, declines to a rate of between 2% to 5% per year in the elderly. Rates of remodeling in trabecular bone are proportionately higher throughout life and may normally be five to ten times higher than cortical remodeling rates in the adult.

Slide II,3 illustrates some of the events in internal bone remodeling. Both cortical and cancellous bone are constantly remodeled by a specific cycle of cellular activity. Initially, bone is resorbed by osteoclasts both in the cortex and on the trabeculae (1). Bone formation by means of osteoblastic activity occurs on the site of the old resorbed bone (2). The osteoblasts themselves become incorporated into bone as osteocytes (3). Flattened cells line surfaces of bone and probably function similar to osteocytes. Under normal circumstances, the remodeling process of resorption followed by formation is closely coupled and results in no net change in bone mass. A bone metabolic unit (BMU) consists of a group of all the linked cells that participate in remodeling a certain area of bone. It was originally thought that all cells in a BMU originate from a single cell line. Recent work suggests that osteoclasts are derived from the monocyte-macrophage cell line of bone marrow. The origins of the osteoblast and osteocyte are not well understood.

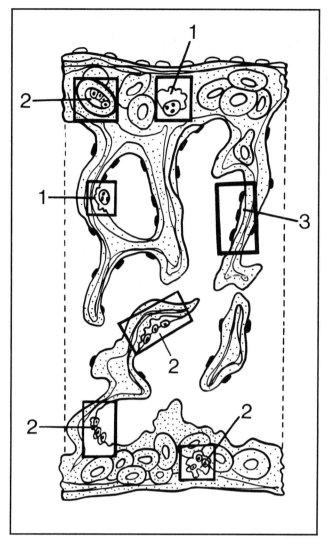

Slide II,3

The dynamics of bone remodeling are nicely illustrated in the microradiograph in Slide II,4. On the left, a thin section of cortical bone is revealed by tetracycline double labeling. Tetracycline is incorporated at sites of active mineralization of bone matrix (concentric circles); by measuring time and distance between deposits, mineralization rates in bone remodeling can be assessed. The darker areas peripherally represent quiescent areas of the osteon. In the corresponding microradiograph on the right, the most newly formed bone (surrounding the haversian canal) is least mineralized and appears dark, while the oldest bone, which is the most highly mineralized (but quiescent from the standpoint of remodeling) in fact appears quite light. This slide demonstrates the heterogeneity of adjacent bone caused by age and the continual internal remodeling of cortical bone.

Cortical bone remodeling depends on a mechanism employing cutting cones (Slide II,5) and is similar to processes in other hard biological tissues. Cutting cones bore holes through the hard bone, leaving tunnels, which seem in cross-section to represent resorption cavities. (See Slide II,4). The head of the cutting cone consists of osteoclasts that resorb the bone. Following the osteoclasts is a capillary loop and osteoblasts to fill in the resorption cavity. By the end of the process, a new osteon has been formed, which is the substance of the cortical bone.

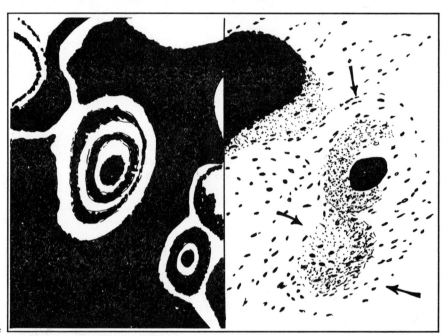

Slide II,4

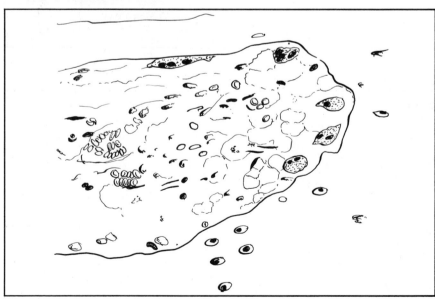

Slide II,5

Bone Metabolism and Homeostasis

Vitamin D Pathway

Vitamin D is a potent calcitrophic hormone. Its primary function is to enhance calcium and phosphorus absorption across the gut and from the bone. Ultraviolet light acting upon the skin transforms 7-dehydrocholesterol into vitamin D_3. One hour of direct sunlight on a caucasian face produces the daily requirement of 400 units. Dark-skinned individuals require more sun exposure. Vitamin D occurs rarely in natural foods (cod liver oil) and consequently is added to some foods as Vitamin D_2 (radiated ergosterol). Vitamin D (2 or 3) is hydroxylated in the liver to 25(OH) vitamin D. Both vitamin D and 25(OH) vitamin D are inactive precursor vitamins. A serum 25(OH) vitamin D level is the best indication of body stores of vitamin D. In the presence of parathyroid hormone (PTH), the mitochondria of the kidney's proximal tubules further hydroxylate the 25(OH) vitamin D into the active hormone metabolite $1,25(OH)_2$ vitamin D. In the absence of PTH, 25(OH) vitamin D is hydroxylated to $24,25(OH)_2$ vitamin D. Slide II,6 illustrates the metabolic pathways of vitamin D.

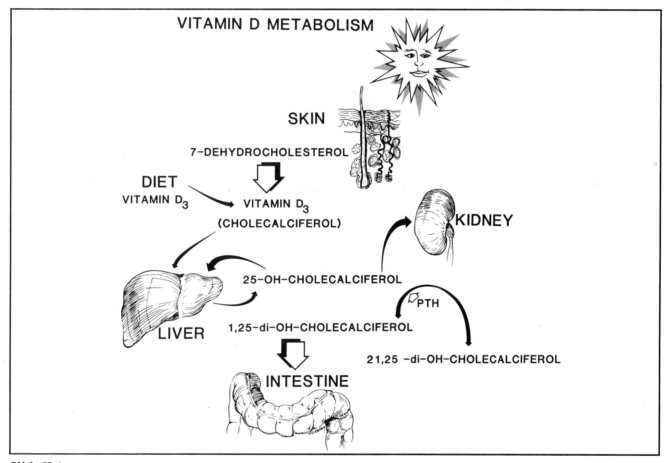

Slide II,6

Calcium Homeostasis

Slide II,7 summarizes calcium homeostasis. Calcium homeostasis depends primarily upon PTH, calcitonin and 1,25(OH)$_2$ vitamin D activity upon the kidney, gut, and bone. Calcium and phosphorus absorption across the intestine and calcium and phosporus resorption from bone are actively enhanced by 1,25(OH)$_2$ vitamin D. PTH directly augments calcium resorption from the kidney and bone in conjunction with 1,25(OH)$_2$ vitamin D and indirectly enhances calcium absorption across the gut by stimulating the conversion of 25(OH) vitamin D to 1,25(OH)$_2$ vitamin D. Calcitonin's primary function is to decrease calcium resorption from bone by decreasing osteoclast activity and number.

In the face of a low serum calcium ion level, PTH is released and stimulates 1,25(OH)$_2$ vitamin D production. Calcium is resorbed from bone and absorbed across the gut, all leading to an elevation of serum calcium. When calcium levels are too high, such as after a large dairy meal in children, PTH is turned off and all the above activities are curtailed. In excessive hypercalcemia, calcitonin is released, further curtailing baseline osteoclastic resorptive activity and thus lowering serum calcium.

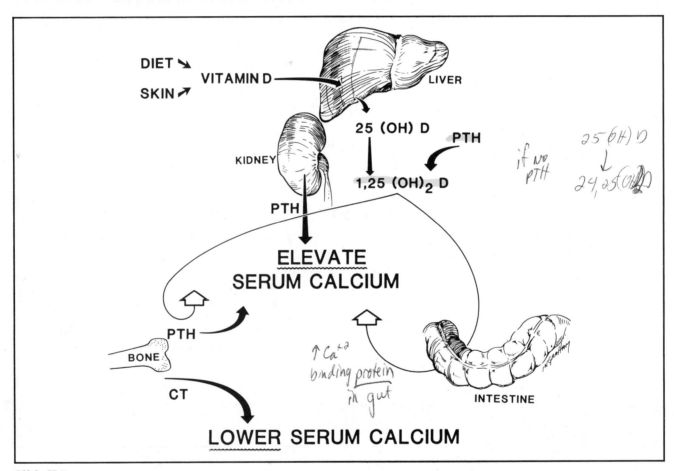

Slide II,7

PTH — directly stimulates osteoblasts initially, which release mediators & subsequently stimulate osteoclasts

Supplement c̄ regular(plain) Vit D to leave regulatory mechanisms intact
if gut problems/etc - use 25 OH Vit D

Calcium Nutritional Requirements

Slide II,8 depicts calcium requirements by age. Proper calcium nutrition is critical to bone maintenance. Chronic mild deficiency will lead to a negative calcium balance and gradual loss of bone mass. In young individuals, approximately 15% to 25% of ingested calcium is absorbed. In elderly persons, this percentage declines; consequently, they require more dietary calcium to achieve the same net calcium transport across the gut. Similarly, augmented dietary calcium may be necessary during the adolescent growth spurt, early adulthood when maximum bone mass is being achieved, during pregnancy, and especially during lactation.

The following table highlights the calcium requirement by age and activity level.

GROUP	DAILY ELEMENTAL CALCIUM REQUIREMENTS
Youth (0-10 years)	500-700 mg
Growth spurt to young adult (10-25 years)	1300 mg
Adult (25-30 years)	750 mg
Postmenopausal	1500 mg
Pregnancy	1500 mg
Lactation	2000 mg

Age-Related Changes Of Bone Mass

Slide II,9 illustrates the relationship among age, bone mass, and sex. Much anabolic skeletal activity occurs during the adolescent growth spurt. Early in adolescence, the skeleton undergoes rapid longitudinal growth with only moderate increase in mineral content. An increase in cortical porosity offsets the increase in periosteal and endosteal apposition. Increased bone turnover provides some of the minerals needed for the new bone. Not until late adolescence, when longitudinal growth slows, does bone mineral content rapidly increase. Bone mass peaks after skeletal maturity some time during the third decade.

In the period between the onset of adolescence and skeletal maturity, dietary habits and hereditary factors play a large role in determining the ultimate size of the bone mineral bank. The size of this bank stays nearly constant throughout most of adult life, with the body redistributing its assets according to structural needs until the fifth decade, when it begins to decline. Sex differences in bone loss are dramatic. Bone mass decreases more rapidly in women than in men, and at locally variable rates throughout the skeleton. Evidence from kinetic studies indicates that after age 40, formation rates remain constant while resorption rates increase. Over several decades, the skeletal mass may be reduced to 50% of that at age 30.

In the decade after age 40, men lose only about 0.5% to 0.75% of bone mass yearly, while women lose bone at more than twice that rate (1.5% to 2% a year). Following menopause, the rate of bone loss in some women may temporarily approach 3% a year.

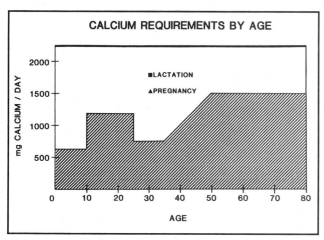

Slide II,8

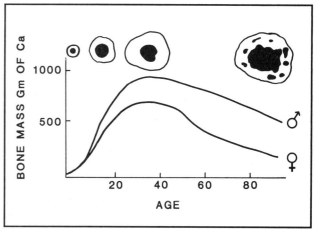

Slide II,9

↓ Mg leads to hypoparathyroidism
so if ↓ Ca⁺ᵈ, give continuous low infusion of Mg if
have low Mg

Metabolic Bone Disease

Metabolic bone diseases are generalized disorders of skeletal homeostasis, and comprise some of the most common and the most esoteric disorders seen by the orthopaedist. While great progress has been made over the past decade in the understanding of metabolic bone disease, diagnostic difficulty has resulted in great confusion, so basic definitions are essential. Osteopenia is a generic term used to describe the radiographic picture of "washed-out" bone. The term osteopenia conveys no information about the underlying etiology of the condition. Osteoporosis, on the other hand, is a more specific term referring to a state of decreased mass per unit volume (density) of normally mineralized bone matrix. The bone is qualitatively normal, but there is less of it when compared to normal age- and sex-matched controls. Osteomalacia (soft bones, or adult rickets) must be considered in the differential diagnosis of osteopenia. Osteomalacia is a qualitative disorder of bone metabolism and refers to an increased, normal, or decreased mass of insufficiently mineralized bone matrix. These relationships are depicted in the upper frame of Slide II,10.

Although plain radiographs are useful in the initial evaluation of osteopenia, they are the least sensitive method of assessing bone mass. Bone mass must be decreased by 40% to 50% before osteopenia can be detected on plain radiographs. During the past decade, noninvasive radiographic and radioisotopic techniques have been developed to determine skeletal mass. These techniques are more precise, sensitive and safe, although the accuracy of the different techniques may vary as much as 20%. Actual quantitation of bone mass *in vivo* helps to establish the severity of bone loss in an osteopenic patient and serves as a baseline for evaluation or therapy. Techniques available for noninvasive quantitation of bone mass include single-photon absorptiometry of the forearm, dual-photon absorptiometry of the lumbar spine, and quantitative computed tomography of the lumbar spine for evaluation of vertebral trabecular bone density. These noninvasive *in-vivo* techniques are of no value in determining the quality of bone matrix mineralization. They cannot be used to differentiate between osteoporosis and osteomalacia, the two most common generic osteopenic conditions. The most sensitive tool available for evaluating the quality of bone matrix (osteoid) mineralization, and thus for determining the presence of osteomalacia, is a full-thickness transiliac bone biopsy that includes both the cortical and trabecular bone of the iliac crest. The results of this biopsy are illustrated in the lower frame of Slide II,10 (arrow). Iliac bone biopsy allows quantitative evaluation of bone formation, resorption, cell populations, and matrix mineralization.

Osteomalacia

Osteomalacic syndromes are of diverse etiology and are characterized pathophysiologically by a failure of normal mineralization of bone matrix (osteoid). It is incorrect to say that the bones are demineralized, as that process does not occur *in vivo*. The body cannot dissolve the mineral out of bone. Demineralization implies that the bones were normally mineralized and then subsequently lost calcium and phosphorus. If the serum calcium falls below normal, PTH is released and osteoclastic bone resorption occurs, with dissolution of both organic matrix and mineral. How then does osteomalacia occur? Osteomalacia results from the failure of mineralization of the newly formed osteoid. Albright understood this quite well when he inferred that any condition causing the serum calcium-phosphorus product to remain below 30 would lead to rickets in the child and to osteomalacia in the adult. Albright's inference helps us to understand the two major causes of osteomalacia: disorders of vitamin D metabolism and renal disease.

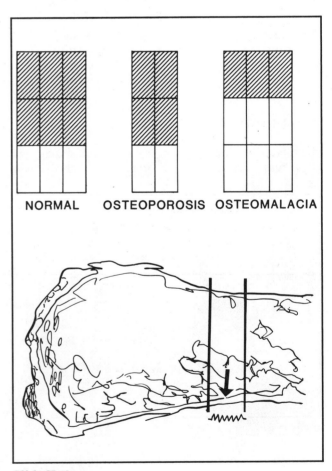

NORMAL   OSTEOPOROSIS   OSTEOMALACIA

Slide II,10

Abnormalities of the Vitamin D Pathway Regardless of the underlying cause, be it true vitamin D deficiency, malabsorption, increased peripheral utilization (anticonvulsants), renal osteodystrophy, or the rare enzymatic deficiency of the final converting enzyme, $1,25(OH)_2$ vitamin D in the kidney, all vitamin D pathway abnormalities manifest decreased circulating levels of the active hormone, $1,25(OH)_2$ vitamin D, and ultimately a decreased serum calcium-phosphorus product. The result is a mineralization product insufficient to allow proper mineralization of any newly formed bone matrix. An undecalcified transiliac bone biopsy reveals both an increased thickness in the osteoid seams and an increased trabecular bone surface area. Tetracycline labeling will reveal a decrease in the mineral apposition rate and smudging of the label, a diagnostic and pathognomonic feature of osteomalacia. In addition, evidence of secondary hyperparathyroidism (osteitis fibrosa or peritrabecular fibrosis) can be seen. Secondary hyperparathyroidism always accompanies the vitamin D pathway abnormalities, and it represents the body's normal homeostatic response to a low serum calcium. The histologic findings in hyperparathyroidism are demonstrated in the right side of Slide II,11. Note that the marrow is densely fibrotic in focal areas near the bone, as the result of PTH stimulation. Note also the increased number of osteoclasts in a given field.

Hypophosphatemic Conditions (Renal tubular conditions—Vitamin D Resistance) Numerous conditions affect the renal tubules and all cause impaired tubular phosphate reabsorption. The most common condition is familial, or x-linked dominant hypophosphatemic vitamin D-resistant rickets. Other examples include the Fanconi syndromes, with additional loss of glucose or amino acids or both; the renal tubular acidosis syndromes; and the hypophosphatemic osteomalacia that may accompany fibrous dysplasia, neurofibromatosis or other soft-tissue tumors producing hypophosphatemic factors. All of these conditions are described as being vitamin D resistant, since even massive doses of vitamin D fail to correct the condition. The major defect is not in the vitamin D pathway, but in the body's ability to conserve phosphorus. The calcium-phosphorus product is insufficient to support mineralization of newly formed osteoid and the result is osteomalacia. In these conditions, however, there is no secondary hyperparathyroidism, as the serum calcium is characteristically normal. Hence, the histologic picture is that of pure osteomalacia with widened osteoid seams, impaired osteoid mineralization, and increased total bone surface area covered by unmineralized or hypomineralized matrix. Peritrabecular fibrosis or osteitis fibrosa (both expressions of marrow stimulation by PTH) are absent, and osteoclast numbers are diminished. These histologic changes are well demonstrated in the undecalcified section at the left of Slide II,11, which can be contrasted to the right frame. In addition to the two major categories of osteomalacia just discussed, several other minor ones are worth mention.

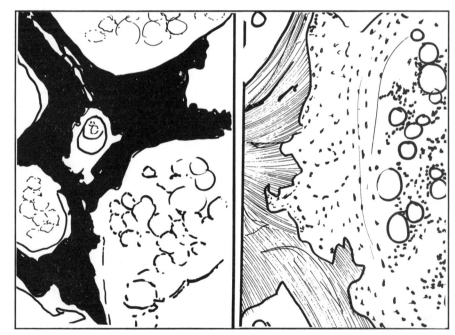

Slide II,11

Hypophosphatasia This disorder results from a genetic error in the synthesis of alkaline phosphatase and is transmitted as an autosomal recessive trait. A decreased level of serum alkaline phosphatase is noted in bone, cartilage, liver, intestinal mucosa and kidney. Increased serum and urine concentrations of phosphoethanolamine are found in both affected individuals and in asymptomatic carriers of this trait. Changes are usually manifested early in life; growth retardation, failure to thrive, irritability, fever, vomiting and signs of increased intracranial pressure are characteristic. Subsequently, individuals may develop alterations in the bones indistinguishable from those of rickets. A milder form occurs in adolescents and adults and may present with early loss of teeth or mild osteomalacia. Alkaline phosphatase is thought to be an important enzyme produced by the osteoblast in preparing the bone matrix for mineralization. Histologically, this type of osteomalacia is indistinguishable from osteomalacia secondary to vitimin D abnormalities (shown in Slide II,11).

Miscellaneous Disorders The ingestion of heavy metals, such as cadmium, berylium, and aluminum may produce an osteomalacic syndrome. Aluminum-caused osteomalacia may be seen as a manifestation of aluminum hydroxide gel ingestion (phosphate binders) by patients with renal osteodystrophy. The aluminum can be located by special stains in the enlarged osteoid seams. Excessive sodium fluoride and diphosphonate ingestion can also cause an osteomalacic syndrome.

Renal Osteodystrophy

Perhaps the most frequently encountered rachitic and osteomalacic state today is renal osteodystrophy. Chronic glomerular renal disease resulting in renal insufficiency, azotemia and acidosis has a profound effect on the skeletal system. The changes include rickets or osteomalacia, osteitis fibrosa cystica, osteosclerosis and metastatic calcification. The extraordinary clinical picture produced by these combinations is termed renal osteodystrophy. The pathogenesis of the bone changes in renal osteodystrophy is complex and is depicted on Slide II,12. In a patient with chronic renal disease, glomerular damage may be so severe that urea cannot be excreted, leading to uremia. If a molecule as small as urea cannot be excreted, phosphate retention also occurs, producing hyperphosphatemia. In addition, the tubular damage in uremia is almost always sufficient to cause reduced synthesis of $1,25(OH)_2$ vitamin D. Hyperphosphatemia alone results in suppressed synthesis of $1,25(OH)_2$ vitamin D. Hyperphosphatemia and the reduced amount of the vitamin cause a profound reduction in the gastrointestinal absorption of calcium. Hypocalcemia results, which not only leads to rickets and osteomalacia, but also induces secondary hyperparathyroidism and the characteristic bone changes classically known as osteitis fibrosa cystica. Because serum calcium increases as a result of the secondary hyperparathyroidism, the serum calcium and phosphate product may exceed the critical solubility product for these two ions and result in ectopic calcification. For reasons not known, approximately 20% of patients with

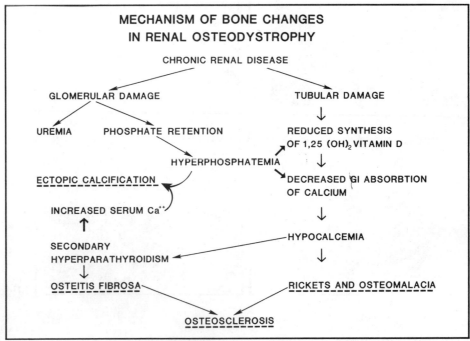

Slide II,12

[handwritten notes] Calitonin = ? urine Ca, = opposes PTH → but lowers serum PO4 just like PTH

Ca is low but within nl limits

renal failure, secondary hyperparathyroidism (osteitis fibrosa) and rickets or osteomalacia may develop a patchy osteosclerosis. In addition to an elevated blood urea nitrogen (BUN) and creatinine, in these 20% of patients the serum calcium is usually normal or low and the serum inorganic phosphate markedly elevated. Fecal calcium is increased, phosphate diminished and PTH levels are almost invariably increased. Aluminum hydroxide gel administration may contribute to the osteomalacia.

The bone changes resulting from these marked aberrations in physiology consist of rickets or osteomalacia, hyperparathyroidism, osteosclerosis, and metastatic calcification. The latter occurs in four characteristic sites: the conjunctivae; the media of the larger blood vessels; the periarticular regions; and in the skin.

Clinical and Radiographic Manifestations Of Osteomalacia

The clinical diagnosis of osteomalacia in the adult is often considerably more difficult to establish than that of rickets in a child. Part of this difficulty lies in the relatively mild, slowly progressive alterations produced by the syndrome.

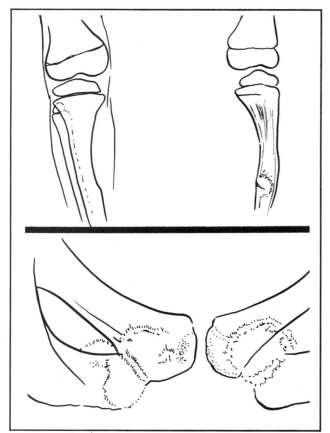

Slide II,13 *Phosphate wasting disorder: Vit D. deficiency*

On radiographs of osteomalacia (Slide II,13), the findings are those of osteopenia. However, pathognomonic features may be found. As seen in the upper frame of Slide II,13, the radiolucent transverse defects are often on the convex sides and are imcomplete. They are frequently found on the medial side of the neck of the femur, the ischial and pubic rami, the ribs, and the scapula. These occasionally become the site of a true fracture, presumably as a result of torsional, tensile or shearing stress in the weakened area. Histologic examination of the pseudofracture site shows a localized increase in deposition of osteoid with very poor mineralization of trabeculae or cortex. The bone scan is a sensitive diagnostic tool for recognizing these fractures. Osteomalacia should be considered in the differential diagnosis whenever symmetrical bone pain and tenderness are present. In osteoporosis, the laboratory data are often normal.

In osteomalacia, the laboratory data are characteristically abnormal, as noted below:

	Vit D Defic.	ED*	VDRR** *(inability to conserve PO4)*	ROD***
Serum Calcium	L or N	L or N	N	L
Serum Phosphorus	L	L	(L)	H
Alkaline Phosphatase	H	H	(L or N)	H
PTH	H	H	N	H
25-OH-D	L	N	N	N
1,25(OH)₂-vit D	L	L	N	L
Urine calc (24 hr)	L	L	N	L

(Ca²⁺ is normal)

* 1,25(OH)₂ D enzyme deficiency.
** Vitamin D-Resistant Rickets.
*** Renal osteodystrophy.

In summary, for most forms of osteomalacia, secondary hyperparathyroidism is a concomitant partner. In secondary hyperparathyroidism, elevated PTH levels are an adaptive and protective physiologic response to low serum calcium levels. In primary hyperparathyroidism, PTH levels are autonomously elevated. The two forms of hyperparathyroidism can be differentiated by serum and urine calcium levels and by mineral apposition rates:

	Primary HPT	Secondary HPT
Serum Calcium	H	L or N
Serum Phosphorus	L	L or N
Alkaline phosphatase	H or N	L or N
Urine Calcium *(low initially →)*	H	L
Osteoclast Activity	L	H
Peritrabecular fibrous tissue	none	present
mineralization	*normal*	*abnormal (defective)*

Clinical and Radiographic Abnormalities of Renal Osteodystrophy

Slide II,14 shows a radiograph of renal osteodystrophy, but the findings are similar to those in osteomalacia or rickets from other causes. There is a characteristic loss of definition of the provisional calcification zone, axial increase in height of the epiphyseal line, and cupping and flaring of the epiphyseal regions, all features observed in patients with vitamin D-deficient or resistant states. Occasionally, slipping at the proximal femoral physis may occur; this phenomenon rarely occurs with conventional rickets and appears to be peculiar to renal osteodystrophy.

Osteopenic Endocrinopathies

In contrast to osteomalacia, a large number of endocrinopathies affect bone formation or resorption and lead to osteopenia. These include parathyroid excess, thyroid hormone excess, Cushing's disease, juvenile onset diabetes mellitus (type I), and estrogen deficiency (Slide II,15). Estrogen supplementation initially decreases bone resorption but does not alter formation, thus leading to mild bone accretions. Following prolonged estrogen administration, formation ultimately

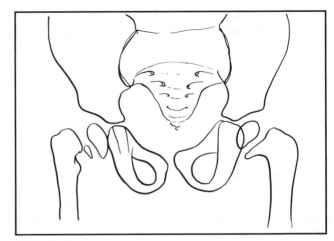

Slide II,14

is decreased so that there is no long-term net mass change. Consequently, the primary effect of estrogen therapy is the maintenance of bone mass.

Calcitonin decreases osteoclastic and osteocytic bone resorption and for the short term enhances bone formation, leading to net bone accretion. In long-term treatment, osteoblastic activity slows and bone mass becomes stabilized.

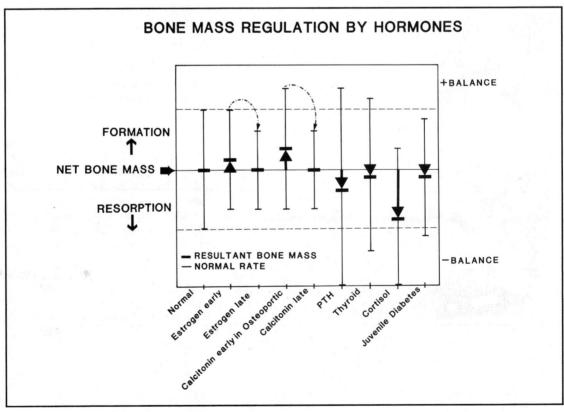

Slide II,15

PTH enhances both bone resorption (osteoclastic activity) and bone formation (osteoblastic activity). Overall metabolism is enhanced and resorption surpasses formation leading to net bone loss. Thyroid hormone excess is similar in effect to excessive PTH but, the degree of hypermetabolism is less. A slow gradual loss of bone mass takes place. Often, thyroid supplementation can lead to prolonged minor bone loss even when given within the normal range, particularly if "high" normal.

Excessive cortisol levels are most deleterious to bone mass. This corticosteroid decreases calcium absorption across the gut, enhances calcium loss from the kidney, inhibits bone formation (especially collagen synthesis), and causes secondary hyperparathyroidism with concurrent enhancement of bone resorption. There is marked loss of bone mass when cortisol levels approach twice normal values. An alternate-day treatment regimen with one day at physiologic levels may be less damaging. Administration of calcium, vitamin D, and hydrochlorothiazide (to prevent renal calcium loss) may counter some of the deleterious effects of cortisol administration.

Juvenile-onset diabetes mellitus (type I) may lead to bone loss. Poorly controlled diabetes mellitus leads to diuresis of calcium. Bone formation is decreased and secondary hyperparathyroidism compensating for urinary calcium loss leads to net bone loss.

Osteoporosis

With age, everyone loses bone mass, but not everyone has osteoporosis. This distinction relates to the amount and nature of the bone loss. Physiologically, the net cortical thickness decreases with age (Slide II,16 left). In women at menopause, bone loss becomes most marked (II,16 right). Regardless of age at the onset of menopause, at that time a woman begins to lose 2% trabecular bone mass per year. Multiple factors contribute to the development of osteoporosis. These include decreased activity, a calcium-deficient diet, inherited characteristics, and factors related to childbirth, premature menopause, and alcoholism.

Estrogen deficiency is directly implicated in the etiology of osteoporosis. Although postmenopausal women produce estrogen, the levels are below those of premenopausal women and age-matched men. Twenty percent of postmenopausal women have a marked paucity of estrogen.

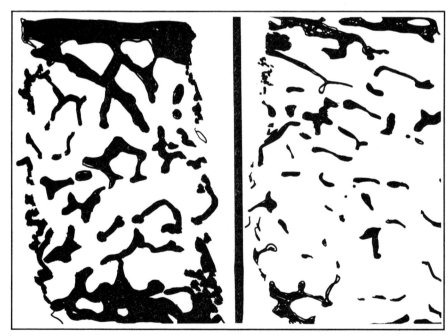

Slide II,16

Slide II,17 illustrates current concepts of calcium metabolism in osteoporosis. Osteoporosis, at least in one early stage, has been found to have increased bone resorption over bone formation (lower right-hand corner of the slide). Later, senile bone with very little cellular activity can be found. Hypermetabolic stages, as well as a stage including increased osteoid, have also been identified in osteoporosis.

Traditionally, most serum laboratory studies are normal, including serum calcium and phosphorus. Following a recent fracture, the alkaline phosphatase may be temporarily elevated. Urinary calcium is frequently decreased, particularly in patients with a long history of reduced dietary calcium intake.

The primary consequences of bone loss are hip, Colle's and vertebral fractures. Calcium intake has been identified as a key factor in fracture incidence. Individuals ingesting physiologic levels of calcium have one-fourth to one-third the rate of hip fractures experienced by individuals with low calcium intake. Calcium prophylaxis appears to be warranted, particularly in high-risk individuals.

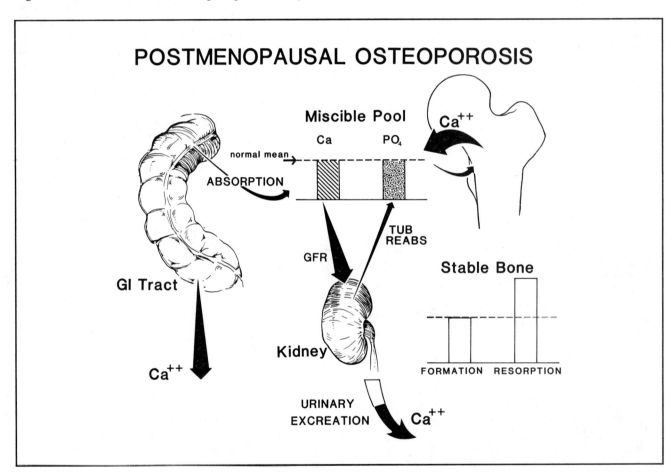

Slide II,17

Treatments of osteoporosis have had variable success for two reasons: inaccurate diagnosis, and insufficient understanding of the disease process. Slide II,18 illustrates the various treatments recommended for osteoporosis. Phosphate and diphosphonate have been unsuccessful, as they only enhance bone loss. Calcium, physiologic vitamin D, calcitonin plus calcium, estrogen plus calcium, and mild exercise appear to decrease bone resorption and to mineralize osteoid, but do not increase total bone mass. No estrogen receptors have been found in bone cells, so estrogen presumably has an indirect effect on bone, possibly via endogenous calcitonin stimulation. The continued use of these agents will decrease or stop postmenopausal bone loss for at least the first decade after menopause, and thereafter with decreasing effectiveness.

Sodium fluoride given with calcium, and physiologic vitamin D increase bone formation and stabilize hydroxyapatite crystals. Estrogen and calcitonin administration may enhance this process. Unfortunately, fluoritic bone is histologically abnormal. High levels of fluoride produce brittle bones and increase fractures.

While low levels of activity can decrease bone loss, extensive exercise can augment bone mass in the highly stressed bone. Recently, the management of osteoporosis has been directed at prevention. Physiologic calcium, vitamin D, estrogen and appropriate exercise would seem to limit the natural loss of bone.

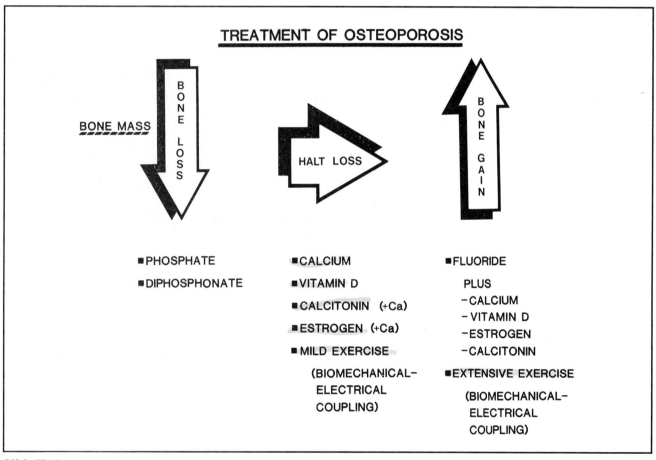

Slide II,18

Paget's Disease

In l877, Sir James Paget described a bone disease which he termed "osteitis deformans." Autopsy studies have yielded a 3% prevalence in a population age 40 and older and a 10% prevalence in those patients over 90 years old. The disease is more common in England, Australia, New Zealand, and Germany than elsewhere; it is rare in Scandanavia. In 15% to 25% of cases, a familial incidence has been clearly documented. Clinically, a large number of patients are asymptomatic.

The radiographic features of Paget's disease are illustrated in Slide II,19 left. The distal tibia demonstrates the advancing osteolytic front, whereas thickening of the cortices with loss of normal architectural configuration and deformity is seen in the proximal portion of the tibia.

In the initial phase of Paget's disease, the dominant feature is osteoclasis (Slide II,19 right). In the active phase, both osteoclastic destruction and osteoblastic formation (the two phases of bone remodeling) occur in the same area of the bone. Pagetic bone is remodeled at a higher rate than that required by the mechanical forces applied to it. The inactive or "burnt out" phase is characterized by a dense mosaic bone pattern and little cellular activity. Often all three phases of Paget's disease may be seen in the same bone biopsy specimen.

Multiple resorbing and forming surfaces are characteristic of pagetoid bone. This chaotic process leads to reorganization of the large plates of oriented lamellar bone into small areas of disorganized bone segments (Slide II,19).

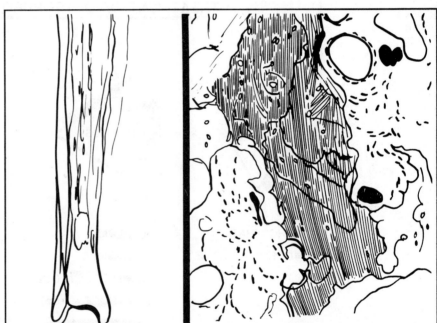

Slide II,19

In a biopsy of a pagetoid vertebral body (Slide II,20 top), multiple resorbing lacunae are visualized. When the same slide is reviewed under polarized light (Slide II,20 bottom), there is clear evidence for disorganization of the collagen fibrils. The consequence of disorganization of the matrix is the enhanced brittle nature of the pagetoid matrix and the high incidence of pathologic fracture and deformity. Fractures heal in pagetic bone at a slower rate than normal because the remodeling process never restores the strength of the fracture site to that of normal bone.

Besides the classic radiographic and morphologic characteristics of Paget's disease, the hypermetabolic state gives rise to scintiphotographic and chemical abnormalities. Alkaline phosphatase, a marker of bone formation, and urinary hydroxyproline, an indicator of bone resorption, are both elevated in active Paget's disease, reflecting the coupling that exists between osteoblastic bone formation and osteoclastic bone resorption.

The etiology of Paget's disease is unknown. Therefore, current treatment is directed at controlling the disorder. Three agents have been utilized successfully: calcitonin, diphosphonate, and mithramycin.

Calcitonin decreases bone resorption, as demonstrated microscopically by a return toward a more normal morphology. Diphosphonate curtails both formation and resorption of bone. Unlike calcitonin, which enhances fracture repair, diphosphonate produces osteoid accumulation. Following long-term therapy, diphosphonate may impair fracture union. Mithramycin is a chemotherapeutic agent that can rapidly decrease pagetoid activity. Although the risk of toxicity is greater compared to calcitonin and diphosphonate administration, mithramycin is very effective in treating pending paraplegia and forms of Paget's disease recalcitrant to the other agents.

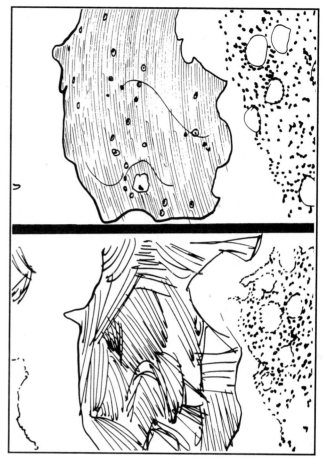

Slide II,20

Bone Repair

Fracture healing or repair may be conveniently described as consisting of five stages: l) impact; 2) inflammation; 3) soft callus; 4) hard callus; and 5) remodeling. The first stage occurs at the moment of impact and lasts until energy is completely dissipated. The stage of inflammation begins at this point and lasts until cartilage or bone formation occurs. This stage is marked by disruption of the blood supply, hemorrhage, and formation of a hematoma. As seen in Slide II,21, bone necrosis occurs at the ends of the fracture fragments, with cellular release of lysosomal enzymes and other by-products of cell death. The first cells to arrive at a fracture site are inflammatory cells, primarily polymorphonuclear neutrophils and macrophages. Fibroblasts appear next to produce collagen in the fracture hematoma. The fracture hematoma is rapidly replaced by granulation tissue consisting of invading capillaries, inflammatory cells, fibroblasts, and collagen. Osteoclasts arrive to remove dead bone at some time during this early period.

The stage of soft callus begins when pain and swelling subside in the extremity and lasts until the bony fragments are united by fibrous or cartilaginous tissue or both. The end of this stage corresponds roughly to when the fragments are no longer movable. This period is marked by increased vascularity of the fracture callus, as shown in Slide II,22. Slide II,23 illustrates the stage of soft callus showing abundant new cartilage formation stained red. Subperiosteal new bone formation begins, and chondroblasts appear in the callus between bone fragments.

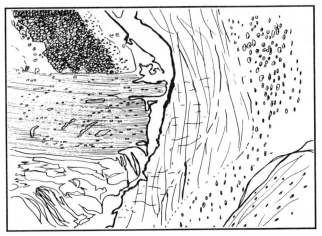

Slide II,21

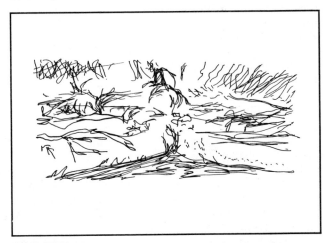

Slide II,22

Hematoma – not necessarily felt to be good anymore

I Injury

II Inflammatory

III Repairative – vasc invasion
pleuripotential cells local tissue periosteum endosteum
  – chondroblasts
  – osteoblasts
  – fibroblasts

IV Remodeling

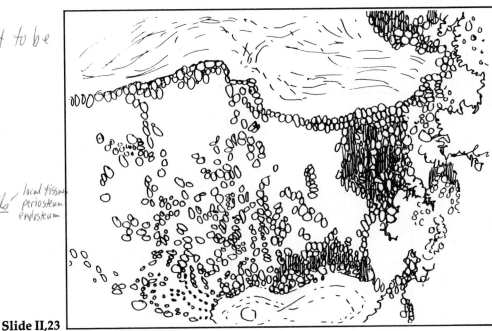

Slide II,23

The stage of hard callus may last three to four months; the end of this stage corresponds to the point when the fracture is clinically and radiographically healed. The callus converts from fibrocartilaginous tissue to fiber bone. Slide II,24 demonstrates the stage of hard callus, showing abundant new bone formation. Some cartilage is still seen. During remodeling, the last stage of fracture healing, fiber bone slowly converts to lamellar bone, and the medullary canal is reconstituted.

Three types of fracture healing have been described. Endochondral fracture healing consists of an initial phase of cartilage formation, followed by new bone formed upon the calcified cartilage template. In membranous fracture healing, bone is formed directly from the mesenchymal tissue without an intervening cartilaginous stage. The typical fracture exhibits both endochondral and membranous bone formation, with the former dominant between the fracture gaps and the latter dominant subperiosteally.

The third type of fracture repair, primary bone healing, occurs without the formation of a visible callus and is seen with rigid internal fixation. The fracture site is bridged by direct haversian remodeling, which is almost a direct osteon-to-osteon hookup. Cutting cones extend across the fracture site and enter the other fragment. Osteoclasts are in the forefront of the cutter heads and remove bone, while osteoblasts trail behind laying down new bone, as shown in Slide II,25. In certain aspects primary bone healing consists of bone remodeling only; that is, there are no histologically discernible stages of inflammation, soft callus, or hard callus.

Four biochemical stages of fracture repair have been described: 1) the mesenchymal stage in which fibroblasts, chondroblasts, and scavenger cells predominate and types I, II, and III collagen are synthesized; 2) the chondroid stage in which cartilage and type II collagen predominate; 3) the chondro-osteoid stage in which calcified bars, primary spongiosa, and types I and II collagen predominate; 4) the osteogenic stage in which there is a progressive shift from primary to secondary spongiosa and type I collagen predominates.

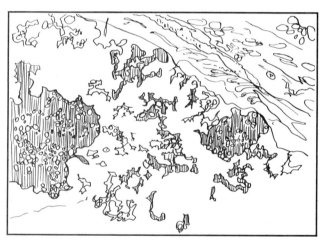

Slide II,24

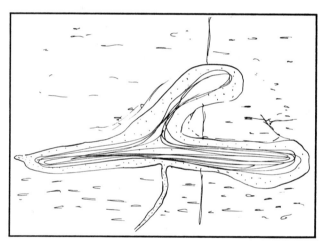

Slide II,25

Healing
① 1° Bone Healing
② External callus
③ 1° Internal Callus
④ 2° Late Internal Callus

Influences on healing
1. Blood Supply
2. Apposition - need 2 bone ends (osteoinduction) eg Adult amputees don't overgrow at bone ends c̄ compression
3. Immobilization, to a certain degree
   (O₂ tension, pH
Signals { BMP (humeral factors)
{ electrical properties (negative charge
4. time

The vascular response to fracture takes place in three phases:phase I (0 to 1 week), local reduction in blood flow rate; phase II (1 to 4 weeks), elevated blood flow rate; phase III (5 to 8 weeks), decreased blood flow rate back to normal levels. Slide II,26 shows blood flow at a fracture site, as determined by an I125-labeled 4-iodoantipyrine washout technique. Blood flow reaches a peak and then progressively decreases.

Profound changes in oxygen tension occur in the fracture callus. As shown in Slide II,27, oxygen tension is very low in the fracture hematoma, low in newly formed cartilage and bone, and highest in fibrous tissue. Oxygen tension in callus fiber bone remains low until the fracture is healed. Despite the great ingrowth of capillaries into the fracture callus, the increase in cell proliferation is such that the cells exist in a state of hypoxia. This hypoxic state could be favorable for bone formation, as *in vitro* bone growth optimally occurs in a low-oxygen microenvironment.

Electric phenomena in bone consist of endogenous signals arising in bone and exogenous signals applied to bone. Two types of endogenous signals have been described: 1) stress-generated potentials that are not dependent on cell viability because they arise from the organic component of bone when it is mechanically stressed; 2) bioelectric potentials that are induced in areas of active bone growth and repair and are dependent on cell viability, but not on mechanical stress. Bioelectric potentials recorded from the surface of a fracture callus are strongly negative throughout the healing process.

Electricity in various forms to treat nonunion is being used at present in the United States and, to a smaller extent, in other parts of the world. Results indicate that the use of electricity, given the proper electric current and voltage and adequate patient compliance, results in the same healing rate in the treatment of nonunion as does bone graft surgery. It has not been demonstrated, however, that electricity can significantly accelerate fresh fracture healing, as apparently electricity converts fibrous tissue at the fracture site to bone rather than inducing more callus formation.

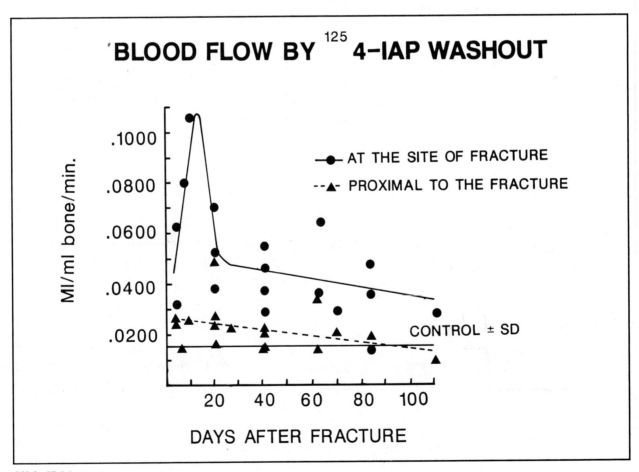

Slide II,26

Factors Influencing Fracture Repair

Fracture healing may be influenced by local and systemic factors. The functional use of the fractured bone, such as provided by a weight-bearing cast or cast brace, promotes healing. The load on the fractured bone does not seem to be important; rather, the functional use of the limb during healing would seem to be the key factor.

Rigid plating may shield the bone from stress and alter its blood supply during remodeling, causing cortical thinning and osteoporosis. The beneficial effect of compression plating is to reduce the fracture gap, thus promoting primary bone healing. Fractures stabilized by plates generally heal by endosteal callus. Fixation of fractures by intramedullary devices damages the medullary blood supply and prevents endosteal callus formation.

Induction

During the process of fracture healing or bone regeneration, certain cells that possess osteogenic potential are stimulated to form bone. Some of these cells, such as osteocytes, periosteal cells, and endosteal cells, are capable of forming bone, but at the time of fracture are not actively engaged in osteogenesis. The process by which a cell is stimulated to activate a normally inactive physiologic process is termed "modulation." If, in response to a fracture, primitive mesenchymal cells that do not possess osteogenic potential are induced to become osteoblasts, the process by which this occurs is termed "induction," and the factors or substances that bring about this induction are called "inductors." Possible inductors present in a fracture callus are various products of cell death; oxygen gradient; electric potential; and bone morphogenetic protein and other noncollagenous proteins.

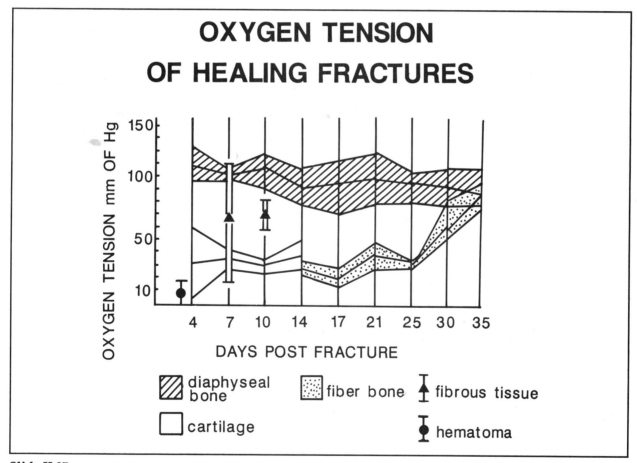

Slide II,27

Nonunion of Bone

The incidence of delayed union is unknown, but the incidence of nonunion has been estimated to be 5% of all long-bone fractures. The bones of the axial skeleton, including skull, vertebral bodies, scapula, ribs, and pelvis rarely exhibit nonunion. In nonunion, new bone formation, cartilage, and fibrous tissue are present and cannot be distinguished from these same tissues as seen in an early-healing callus. (Slide II,28 left side). There is, however, more cartilage and fibrous tissue and less new bone formation in a nonunion than in a healing callus. (Slide II,28 right side) In fibrous nonunion the cartilage and fibrous tissues persist, whereas in healing fractures they are replaced by newly formed bone.

Those nonunions that exhibit significant motion of the fracture for a long time may go on to form a synovial pseudarthrosis at the nonunion site. A fully developed synovial pseudarthrosis is a rather large cavity filled with fluid and lined with a synovial-like membrane. Synovial pseudarthrosis is diagnosed either at the time of surgery or by the aid of 99m-technetium scintigraphy. The vast majority of all nonunions show increased uptake of the radionuclide at the fracture site. In synovial pseudarthrosis, however, a photon-deficient cleft is present between two intense areas of uptake.

Treatment of nonunion is aimed at restarting the regenerating system. Bone graft surgery and electric stimulation in various forms appear to be equally successful in restarting the healing process.

Bone Grafting

Cancellous Autograft Important features of transplant repair include necrosis, revascularization, graft incorporation by host, and creeping substitution. Axhausen used the term "schliechander ersatz," literally translated, "creeping substitution," to describe the process of new tissue invading the dead graft by making new channels or entering along pre-existing channels.

Both cancellous and cortical autogenous transplants have similar histologic features during the first two weeks after transplantation. During the first week, the transplant is the focus of an inflammatory response characterized by vascular buds infiltrating the transplant bed. By the second week, fibrous granulation tissue becomes increasingly dominant in the transplant bed, the number of inflammatory cells decreases, and osteoclastic activity increases. Within the confines of the transplant, osteocytic autolysis occurs. Some peripheral cells are maintained by the passive diffusion of nutrients from the surrounding host soft tissues.

Cancellous bone transplants differ from cortical bone transplants by the rate of revascularization, the mechanism of creeping-substitution repair, and the completeness of repair. Several investigators suggest that revascularization of cancellous transplants may occur within hours after transplantation as the result of end-to-end anastomoses of the host vessels with those of the transplant. Primarily, however, revascularization occurs by gradual host ingrowth into the marrow spaces.

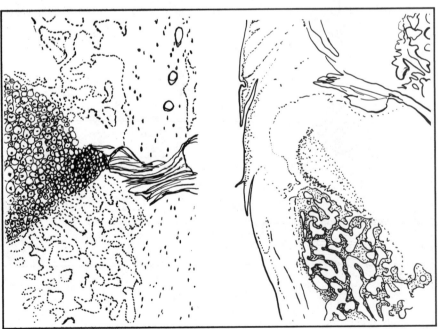

Slide II,28

As the vascular invasion of the cancellous grafts proceeds, primitive mesenchymal cells differentiate into osteogenic cells. Osteoblasts line the edges of dead trabeculae and deposit a seam of osteoid that is annealed to, and eventually surrounds, a central core of dead bone. Radiographically there is an initial increase in the radiodensity. Subsequently, the entrapped cores of necrotic bone are resorbed and a new cortex is reconstituted.

The composite Slide II,29 demonstrates the transition from cancellous bone graft to reconstituted bone. At one week (top panel) the cancellous graft (left) is adjacent to the host cortex, and premature mesenchymal cells are accumulated at the junction. At two weeks (middle panel) new bone formation is noted in both the graft (left) and the host (right). By one year (bottom panel) the autograft has become completely incorporated and has now remodeled into cortex. Little, if any, necrotic bone is present.

Cortical Autograft Cortical bone is frequently transplanted in preference to cancellous bone because of its initial structural properties. Its incorporation and remodeling are quite different from cancellous graft. The cortical graft is not penetrated by blood vessels until the sixth day, and complete revascularization occurs after several months, twice the time span required for cancellous grafts. The delay in revascularization may be attributed to the limited surface area of cortical bone, since vascular penetration of the transplant is primarily the result of peripheral osteoclastic resorption and vascular infiltration.

Spatial analyses of the transplant repair processes in animals shows resorption to be preferentially directed to the peripherally located necrotic haversian system and the interstitial lamellae during the early weeks. Later, resorption of the cortical interior occurs by enlargement of the haversian cavities with no significant removal of necrotic interstitial lamellae. When the appropriate cavity size is attained, resorption ceases and osteoblasts appear and refill the spaces.

Slide II,30 (top) is a photomicrograph demonstrating creeping substitution. Necrotic bone is seen on the left. New bone formation can be noted (to the right) about the haversian canal where necrotic bone has been first resorbed and then replaced by new bone. The bottom half of Slide II,30 is a cross-section of a fibular graft. Most of the cortical graft is necrotic, and numerous resorption cavities can be seen.

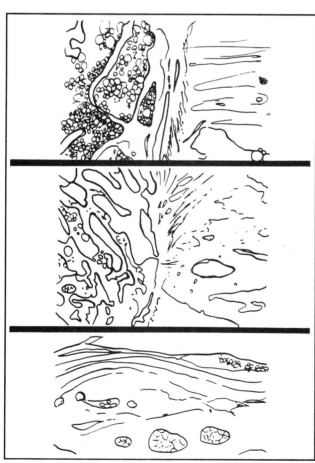

Slide II,29

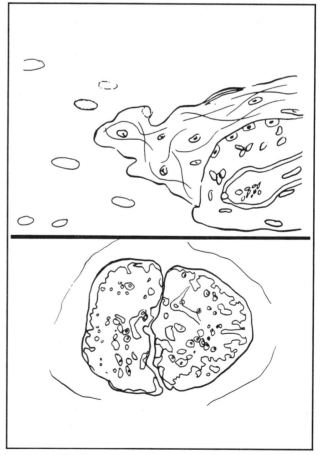

Slide II,30

Genetically Controlled Musculoskeletal Disorders

Biochemical reactions directing growth and development, as well as many structural variations and many degenerative processes treated by orthopaedists are under genetic control. Present estimates suggest that genetic and environmental factors are nearly equal as causes of anomalies in the roughly 5% of babies born with some congenital defect.

There are three major types of genetic control: mendelian inheritance; polygenic inheritance; and chromosomal imbalance. Many genetic diseases are not present or apparent at birth; they may be encountered at any age.

Age of Manifestation of Exemplary Genetic Diseases

CONCEPTION	Chromosomal Rearrangements (miscarriage)
BIRTH	Club Feet
	Dislocated Hip
	Skeletal Dysplasias
CHILDHOOD	Morquio's Syndrome
	Multiple Exostoses
	Vitamin D-Resistant Rickets
	Duchenne's Muscular Dystrophy
ADOLESCENCE	Scoliosis
	Ankylosing Spondylitis
MIDDLE AGE	Dupuytren's contracture

The classic and basic tool of genetics is construction of a pedigree, which is well within the expertise of orthopaedists. Patients with genetic disease sometimes know that it "runs in the family," but often have peculiar notions as to the mechanisms. Sometimes family members are unaware of obvious genetic transmission. It is not enough to ask if other family members have a similar condition. A minimum routine involves three steps: 1) draw the pedigree to include third-degree relatives; 2) name all individuals and inquire about their health; 3) review the pedigree on a subsequent visit. Mendelian and polygenic inheritance and chromosomal rearrangements will be briefly reviewed with particular emphasis on orthopaedic disease.

Mendelian Inheritance

In 1866, Gregor Mendel described the basis of what we now know as mendelian inheritance. These patterns control the transmission of many conditions of the musculoskeletal system. The controlling gene may be on a chromosome unrelated to sex determination (an autosome) or may be on the chromosome controlling sex (sex-linked or x-linked). Four inheritance patterns occur: autosomal dominant; autosomal recessive; sex-linked dominant; and sex-linked recessive.

Autosomal dominant conditions In Slide II,31, typical examples of an autosomal dominant pedigree are given. Note the following genetic features: 1) the heterozygote state manifests the condition; 2) 50% of offspring are affected with no sex preference; 3) normal offspring do not transmit the condition; and 4) male-to-male transmission is required to confirm this pattern of

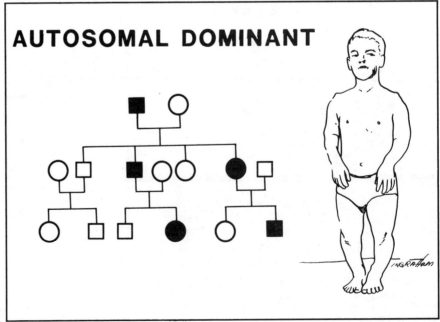

Slide II,31

inheritance. Autosomal dominant conditions often arise as spontaneous mutations. Autosomal dominant conditions are typically nonlethal structural abnormalities. A condition is dominant when expressed clinically even though only one of the two alleles for that gene is abnormal. For example, if half of the structural protein coded by a particular gene is abnormal, then any tissue composed of that protein is likely to be clinically abnormal. The presence of an abnormal gene is an all-or-none phenomenon called "penetrance," while "expressivity" refers to the severity of manifestation of the gene in a particular individual. There may be much variation in the expressivity of an abnormal gene in any particular family. Members of the family who have the abnormal gene may have a range of manifestations. Certain members may have more severe or less severe manifestations than other family members with the abnormal gene.

On the right hand side of Slide II,31 is a young man with achondroplasia, a typical example of an autosomal dominant condition and the most common of the skeletal dysplasias. Other examples of autosomal dominant conditions include: 1) the Marfan syndrome; 2) osteogenesis imperfecta (types I and IV); 3) multiple exostoses; 4) multiple epiphyseal dysplasia; and 5) fibrodysplasia ossificans progressiva.

Autosomal recessive conditions In Slide II,32, a typical example of an autosomal recessive pedigree is shown. Note the following clinical features: 1) the homozygote state manifests the condition; 2) parents are unaffected, but may be related; and 3) 25% of offspring are affected with no sex preference.

Autosomal recessive conditions are classically enzyme defects, "inborn errors of metabolism." "Recessive" means that both of the alleles for that gene must be abnormal to be expressed clinically. If, for example, only one of the alleles that codes for an enzyme is abnormal, then 50% of the enzyme produced will be normal and 50% abnormal. Under most conditions there will still be enough normal enzyme (50%) to catalyze the particular reaction in question, so the disease will not be expressed clinically. This situation is referred to as the heterozygote or carrier state. Single affected persons in a pedigree are common. Parents need not be related to possess common genes. There is little variability in expressivity.

Slide II,32 also shows three children with diastrophic dwarfism, an example of an autosomal recessive condition and a severe chondrodysplasia characterized by short limbs, short stature, severe kyphoscoliosis, joint contractures, hip dysplasia, ear malformation, genu valgum, hitchhiker's thumb, and club feet. A specific enzyme defect has not yet been identified in this condition.

Other autosomal recessive conditions are as follows: 1) most mucopolysaccharidoses including the Hurler and Scheie syndromes, the Sanfilippo syndromes, the Morquio syndromes, and the Maroteaux-Lamy syndrome; 2) homocystinuria; 3) ochronosis; 4) the Ehlers-Danlos syndrome (type V).

Specific enzyme defects have been identified for most of these conditions. The mucopolysaccharidoses can be identified chemically, for example, by the presence of specific mucopolysaccharides that appear in the urine because of the absence or inactivity of a specific degradative enzyme. The clinical manifestations of most mucopolysaccharidoses are caused by abnormal accumulation and storage of mucopolysaccharide in lysosomes of numerous tissues including liver, spleen, skin, cartilage, bone, and brain.

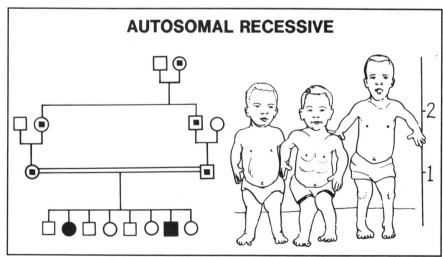

Slide II,32

Sex-linked dominant conditions A typical example of a sex-linked dominant pedigree is seen in Slide II,33. Note the following clinical features: 1) the heterozygote manifests the condition; 2) affected females transmit the x-linked gene to half their daughters and half their sons; 3) affected males transmit x-linked gene to all daughters and to none of their sons; 4) father-to-son transmission does not occur; and 5) males tend to be more severely affected than females. On the right-hand side of Slide II,33, we see family members afflicted with hypophosphatemic vitamin D-resistant rickets (VDRR)

and osteomalacia, the classic sex-linked dominant orthopaedic condition.

Sex-linked recessive conditions A representative sex-linked recessive pedigree is shown in Slide II,34. Note the following clinical features: 1) the heterozygote male is clinically affected, but the heterozygote female is not; 2) the affected male transmits the gene to all daughters, who are carriers, and to none of his sons; and 3) the carrier female transmits the gene to one-half of her daughters, who are carriers, and to one-half of her sons, who are affected.

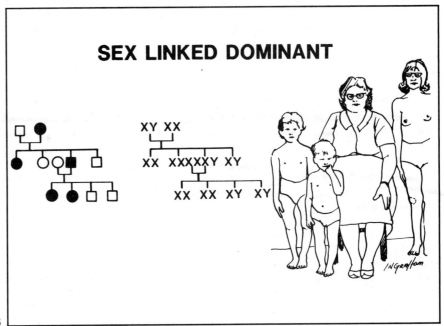

Slide II,33

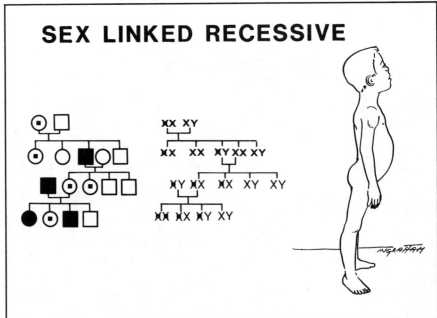

Slide II,34

On the right side of Slide II,34 is a child with Duchenne's muscular dystrophy, the prototype of all muscular dystrophies inherited as a sex-linked (x-linked) recessive condition. Classically, this form of dystrophy affects only males who have inherited the condition from their carrier mothers. A high mutation rate exists, with up to one-third of cases believed to represent mutation. Duchenne's muscular dystrophy typically presents at 3 to 5 years of age with signs of proximal weakness. Independent ambulation is lost, usually by 11 to 13 years of age. Death occurs in the early 20s from cardiomyopathy, or earlier from pulmonary insufficiency. CPK elevation and abnormalities detected by electromyography and muscle biopsy confirm the diagnosis. Many of the *carriers* can be identified by enzymatic abnormalities. Two additional examples of x-linked recessive inheritance include classic hemophilia and Hunter's syndrome (mucopolysaccharidosis II).

Polygenic Inheritance

A second major type of inheritance is polygenic inheritance, which refers to the effects of multiple genes and alleles interacting with environmental factors to influence form and function and incidence of disease. For example, genetic factors appear to control the time of growth-plate closure, but a large number of nutritional and endocrine health factors influence metabolism of the growth plate as well. Height is therefore a polygenic trait. Club feet, congenital dislocation of the hip, and idiopathic scoliosis are examples of polygenic traits. There are important clinical features of polygenic inheritance, some of which are illustrated on the right hand side of Slide II,35.

The likelihood of a condition's occurring in the population can be depicted by a normal Gaussian curve. There is a "threshold" at which a portion of the population may be affected. The threshold reflects both genetic and permissive environmental factors. The level of risk is low. The frequency of recurrence of the same polygenic trait in offspring of unaffected parents is usually in the range of 2% to 6%. There is an increased risk in relatives of those affected. The increased risks are proportional to the genetic similarity. This relationship can be depicted as a shift of the curve on the threshold. The increased risk in relatives is illustrated by idiopathic scoliosis. Thus, scoliosis occurs in approximately 11% of first-degree relatives, 2% of second-degree relatives, and 1% to 2% of third-degree relatives. The threshold of risk is affected by race, sex, and geography. The varying proportions of males to females in polygenic traits illustrate modification by sex.

Risk and severity relate to intrafamily patterns of involvement. Thus, if a parent and child are affected, the odds of subsequent children being affected are greatly increased. The greater the severity, the greater the odds of subsequent children being affected. If the affected individual is of the least-likely affected sex, the odds of subsequent children being affected are generally increased. The inheritance of club foot will be used as a specific example: idiopathic clubfoot occurs in the United States in about 1:1000 births and has a 2:1 male-to-female ratio. It is bilateral in half the children affected. In order to define the recurrence risk for a family, examination must exclude phenocopies (look-alikes), syndromes, mendelian inherited conditions, and chromosomal rearrangements associated with clubfeet.

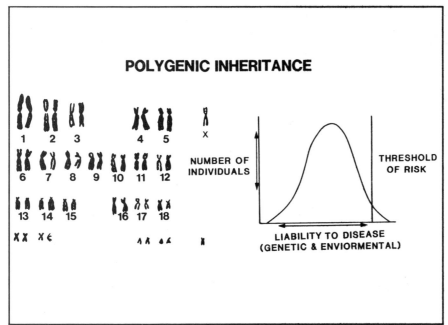

Slide II,35

Chromosome Abnormalities

The last major category of genetic abnormalities comprises chromosomal abnormalities, which are common but often result in miscarrige. About 20% of spontaneous abortions exhibit chromosome abnormalities. About 1% of live births have chromosome abnormalities. The left-hand side of Slide II,35 shows the normal human male karyotype. The normal male has 22 pairs of chromosomes called autosomes and one "X" and one "Y" chromosome. Chromosomes are divided into 7 groups according to morphologic characteristics and are numbered. Chromosome rearrangements occurring in nature are varied and complex. The classic mechanism of producing an extra chromosome (trisomy) or loss of a chromosome (deletion) is failure of separation in the reduction division.

Other types of errors include mosaics (more than one line of cells); translocation (fragmentation of a chromosome with transfer of genetic material to another chromosome); and deletions of parts of chromosomes. Regularity in these accidents allows the delineation of various syndromes, and recent banding techniques have led to increased sophistication in identifying the chromosomes involved. Even so, it is important to realize that large fragments of genetic material are involved, and the clinical syndromes produced are not uniform. The indications for chromosome studies are not precise, but a karyotype analysis should be considered in infants who exhibit the triad of multiple anomalies (especially facial), failure to thrive, and mental retardation. Characteristic associations of chromosome abnormalities that may be seen by orthopaedists include polydactyly in the trisomy-13 syndrome, radioulnar synostosis in the multiple-x syndromes, vertical tali in trisomy-18, and clubfeet in several of the deletion syndromes. The most common chromosome abnormalities with skeletal changes are Down's and Turner's syndromes.

Selected Bibliography

Bone Metabolism and Homeostasis

Boskey A, Posner A: Bone mineral and matrix. Orthopo Clin N Amer 1984.

Glimcher MJ: Composition, structure and organization of bone and mineralized tissues and one mechanism of calcification, in Greep RO, Astwood EB (eds): Handbook of Physiology: Endocrinology. Washington DC, American Physiological Association, 1976, pp 25-116.

Metabolic Bone Disease

Asher M (ed): Orthopaedic Knowledge Update I, Chicago, American Academy of Orthopaedic Surgeons, 1984.

Anast CS, DeLuca F: Pediatric Diseases Related to Calcium. 1980.

Baron R, Vignery A, Horowitz M: Lymphocytes, Macrophages and the Regulation of Bone Remodeling. Bone and Mineral Research Annual 2, 1983; Chap 4, 175.

Barzel US: Osteoporosis. New York, Grune and Stratoon, 1970.

Bourne GH: The Biochemistry and Physiology of Bone, ed 2. New York, Academic Press, 1972.

Ciba Foundation Symposium II (new series): Hard Tissue Growth, Repair and Remineralization. Amsterdam, Associated Scientific Publishers, 1973.

Frost HM: Bone Dynamics in Osteoporosis and Osteomalacia. Springfield, IL, CC Thomas, 1966.

Frost HM: A determinant of bone architect: the minimum effective strain. Clin Ortho 1970; 175:286-292.

Glimcher MJ, Krane SM: The organization and structure of bone and the mechanism of calcification, in Gould BS: Treatise on Collagen, Biology of Collagen. London & New York, Academic Press, 1968, Vol 2; pp 68-251.

Mankin HJ: Rickets, Osteomalacia and Renal Osteodystrophy, Part I and II. J Bone and Joint Surg, 1974; 56A:101-128, 352-386.

Rassmussen H, Bordier P: The Cellular Basis of Metabolic Bone Disease. New Eng J of Med 1973; 289:25-32.

Russell RGG, Smith R: Diphosphonates. J Bone and Joint Surg 1973; 55B:66-86.

Symposium on Metabolic Bone Disease. Ortho Clin of N Amer 1972; November.

Bone Repair

Brighton CT: Principles of fracture healing: part I. The biology of fracture repair, in AAOS Instructional Course Lectures 33. St. Louis, CV Mosby, 1984, chap 3.

Brookes M: The Blood Supply of Bone. New York, Appleton-Century-Crofts, p 270.

Cavadias AN, and Trueta J: An experimental study of the vascular contribution to the callus of fracture. Surg Gynecol Obstet 1965; 120:731.

Lane JM, et al: A temporal study of collagen, proteoglycan, lipid, and mineral constituents in a model of endochondral osseous repair. Metab Bone Relat Res 1979; 1:319.

Laurnen EL, and Kelly PJ: Blood flow, oxygen consumption, carbon dioxide production, and blood calcium and pH changes in tibial fractures in dogs. J Bone Jt Surg 1969; 51A:298.

Panjabi MM, White A III, and Wolf JW Jr: A biomechanical comparison of the effects of constant and cyclic compression on fracture healing in rabbit long bones. Acta Orthop Scand 1979; 50:653.

Pollack SR, et al: Microelectrode studies of stress generated potentials in bone, in Brighton CT, Black J, and Pollack SR (eds):Electrical Properties of Bone and Cartilage. New York, Grune & Stratton, 1979.

Tonna EA, Cronkite EP: Cellular response to fracture studied with tritiated thymidine. J Bone Jt Surg 1961; 43A:352.

Trueta J: The role of vessels in osteogenesis. J Bone Jt Surg 1963; 45B:402.

Urist MR, et al: A bovine low molecular weight bone morphogenetic protein (BMP) fraction. Clin Orthop 1982; 162:219.

Genetically Controlled Disorders

Jackson LG, Schimke RN: Clinical Genetics: A Source Book for Physicians. New York, Wiley, 1979.

McKusik VA: Heritable Disorders of Connective Tissue, ed 3. St Louis, CV Mosby, 1966.

McKusik VA: Mendelian Inheritance in Man: Catalogs of Autosomal Dominant, Autosomal Recessive and X-linked Phenotypes, ed 5. Baltimore, Johns Hopkins, 1978.

Chapter III

Soft Tissue Disorders

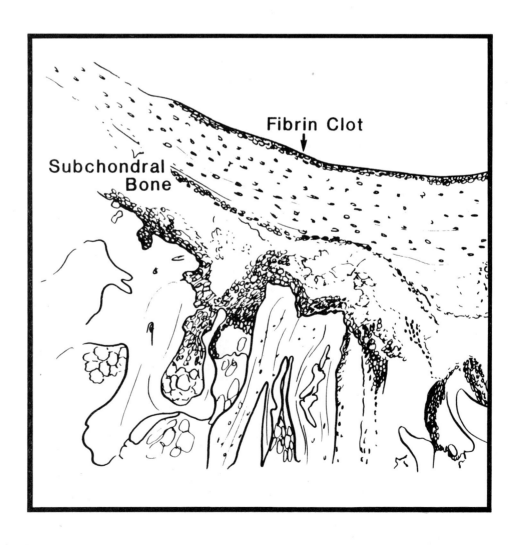

The musculoskeletal soft tissues include cartilage, tendon, intervertebral disc, and muscle. Many clinical problems are related to disturbances in the composition and function of these tissues. Abnormal responses of soft tissues to injury, as well as genetic disorders also present clinical problems. This chapter reviews the biochemical composition and function of articular cartilage, tendon, and intervertebral disc. The repair responses of cartilage and tendon and the degenerative changes in cartilage and intervertebral disc will be discussed. Also discussed will be the genetic disorders osteogenesis imperfecta, Ehlers-Danlos syndrome, and Marfan's syndrome. Finally, neuromuscular disorders and soft-tissue wound repair will be discussed briefly.

Articular Cartilage

Articular cartilage, or hyaline cartilage, is a dense, avascular connective tissue consisting of cells and an abundant extracellular matrix. The matrix forms more than 95% of the tissue and is responsible for the biological and mechanical properties of articular cartilage. As Slide III,1 shows, hyaline cartilage consists primarily of water, whereas other connective tissues and bone contain significantly less water. The matrix macromolecules give hyaline cartilage the ability to maintain its state of hydration and to provide the essential properties of the tissue. Injury or disease of articular cartilage affects the proportions, composition and organization of these macromolecules.

The macromolecular framework of hyaline cartilage is distinguished from other connective tissues by the high content of proteoglycans. Its principal fibrillar collagen is type II collagen. The collagens are a family of distinctive protein macromolecules that give the extracellular framework of connective tissues their tensile strength, as depicted in Slide III,2. Fibrillar collagens consist of amino acid chains called alpha chains in which every third amino acid is glycine. These amino acid chains wrap about each other to form a triple helix, which creates the tropocollagen molecule. A highly ordered arrangement of tropocollagen molecules forms the matrix fibrils of collagen.

As shown in Slide III,3 even the fibrillar collagens differ in composition. Type II collagen is the principal fibrillar collagen of articular cartilage, whereas type I collagen occurs in the dense fibrous tissues and bone. Type II collagen contains more hydroxylysine than type I, and more of its hydroxylysine is glycosylated. Type II collagen characteristically occurs in tissues loaded in compression, whereas type I collagen is more often found in tissues loaded in tension. Currently more than ten collagen types have been described.

Proteoglycans consist of polysaccharide chains of covalently bound protein. In these molecules the carbohydrates form the dominant feature. Cartilage proteoglycans are organized on two levels: subunits or monomers, and aggregates. The subunits consist of thin, central protein cores with multiple chondroitin sulfate and keratan sulfate side chains.

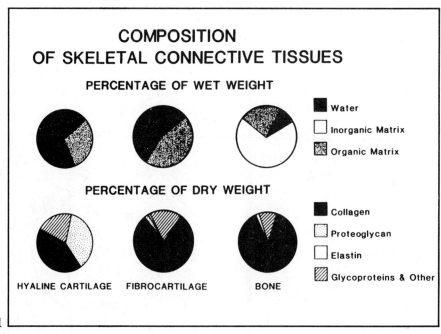

Slide III,1

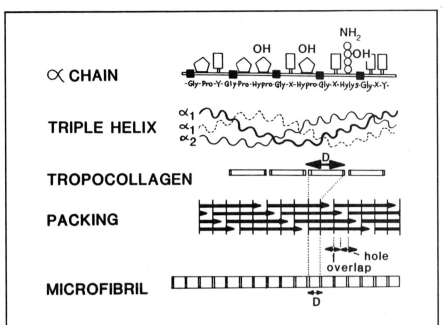

α CHAIN

TRIPLE HELIX

TROPOCOLLAGEN

PACKING

MICROFIBRIL

Slide III,2

COLLAGEN TYPES

INTERSTITIAL

Type	Chains	Native Polymer	Distribution	Hydroxylysine Content Residues/1000	Carbohydrate Content % Hydroxylysine Glycosytate
I.	$[\alpha1(1)]_2\,\alpha2$	FIBRIL	SKIN, TENDON, BONE, MENISCUS ANNULUS	6-8	<20
II.	$[\alpha1(II)]_3$	FIBRIL	HYALINE, CARTILAGE, NUCLEUS PULPOSUS, VITREOUS BODY	20-25	50
III.	$[\alpha1(III)]_3$	FIBRIL	SKIN, BLOOD VESSELS, GRANULATION TISSUE, RETICULIN FIBERS	6-8	15-20

PERICELLULAR AND BASEMENT MEMBRANE

IV.	$[\alpha1(IV)]_2$	BASEMENT LAMINA	KIDNEY GLOMERULI, LENS CAPSULE	60-70	80
V.	$A(\alpha B)_2$ $(\alpha A)_3$ $(\alpha B)_3$	UNKNOWN	CELL SURFACE, PERICELLULAR MATRIX	?	?

Slide III,3

73

Slide III,4 is a diagram showing the proteoglycan subunits as thin core filaments with multiple projecting side chains. These side chains consist of clusters of chondroitin sulfate and keratan sulfate. Keratan sulfate and chondroitin sulfate are called glycosaminoglycans and are depicted in Slide III,5. Their carboxyl and sulfate groups create a string of negative charges which contribute significantly to the behavior of proteoglycans and to their function in articular cartilage.

When minimal or no load is applied to the tissue, the molecules extend themselves until they are restrained by the collagen fibril network. In this extended form they have large molecular domains with relatively low-charge density and low concentrations of chrondroitin sulfate chains. Loading of the tissue forces tissue fluid from the molecular domain, driving the negatively charged chains closer together, as shown in Slide III,6. This action increases their tendency to repel each other and to resist further loading. Relief of the pressure allows the chains to resume their original conformation. Abnormalities in cartilage proteoglycan structure or amount can alter this mechanical property of the cartilage.

Slide III,4

Keratan Sulfate Chains

Chondroitin Sulfate Chains

Protein Core

Keratan Sulfate Rich Region and

Chondroitin Sulfate Rich Region

Hyaluronic Acid Binding Region

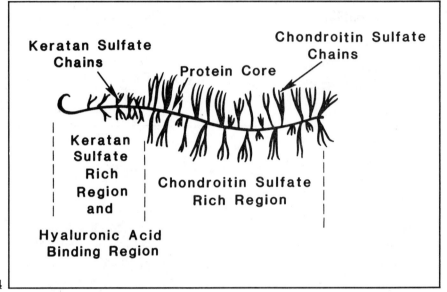

CHONDROITIN 6-SULFATE

KERATAN SULFATE

HYALURONATE

Slide III,5

Slide III,7 illustrates the structure of proteoglycan aggregates. Multiple proteoglycan subunits or monomers bind to hyaluronic acid to form the aggregate. In the cartilage matrix, aggregates immobilize the monomers. The electron photomicrograph shown in Slide III,8 clearly demonstrates the central hyaluronic-acid filament of proteoglycan aggregates as well as the bound subunits.

Notice that most subunits have two distinct segments: a thin segment with few if any side chains that attaches directly to the hyaluronic acid filament and a thick segment with chrondroitin sulfate chains collapsed about the protein core. The thin segment represents the hyaluronic-acid binding region of subunit core protein and some of the keratan-sulfate rich region. The thick segment represents the chrondroitin-sulfate rich region.

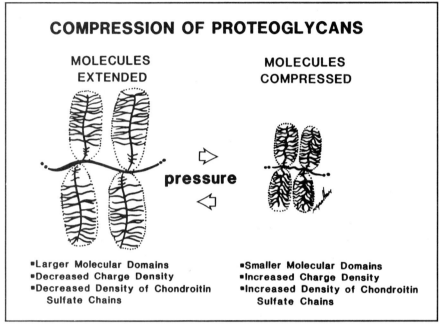

Slide III,6

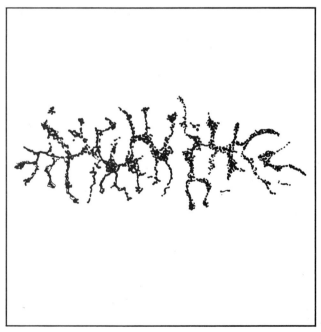

Slide III,7

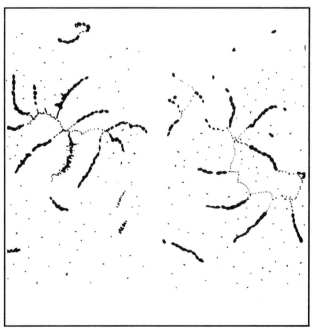

Slide III,8

Slide III,9 lists some of the partially characterized matrix glycoproteins. Glycoproteins generally consist of carbohydrates and protein with the protein forming the dominant feature of the molecules. Functions include mediating the attachment of cells to the matrix, influenc-ing the organization of the matrix macromolecules and perhaps even influencing the behavior of the connective tissue cells. Chondronectin appears to be a significant part of the cartilage matrix and may have a role in attaching chrondrocytes to the matrix.

	Associated Cells	Location	Binding	Molecular Weight
FIBRONECTIN	·FIBROBLASTS ·ENDOTHELIAL CELLS ·OTHERS	·EXTRA CELLULAR MATRIX ·BASEMENT MEMBRANES	·CELL SURFACE ·COLLAGEN ·FIBRINOGEN ·HEPARIN ·HEPARAN SULFATE ·HYALURONIC ACID ·ACTIN ·DNA	420,000 TO 500,000
CHONDRONECTIN	·CHONDROCYTES	·CARTILAGE MATRIX	·CHONDROCYTE SURFACE ·TYPE II COLLAGEN	180,000
OSTEONECTIN	----------	·BONE MATRIX	·COLLAGEN ·HYDROXYAPATITE	32,000
LILAMININ	·EPITHELIAL ·ENDOTHELIAL	·BASEMENT MEMBRANES	·TYPE IV COLLAGEN ·CELL SURFACE ·HEPARIN ·HEPARAN SULFATE	800,000

Slide III,9

As diagrammatically shown in Slide III,10, the three components of proteoglycan aggregates, hyaluronic acid, link protein and the monomers are synthesized within the cell and secreted into the matrix where the aggregate is assembled, just as collagen fibrils are assembled from tropocollagen. Link proteins, represented by the red dots, play an important role in aggregate formation. The link proteins are small polypeptides with a molecular weight of 40,000 to 50,000. In proteoglycan aggregates, they bind simultaneously to the hyaluronic acid binding region of the monomer and to hyaluronic acid. This binding is non-covalent and reversible. Aggregates can form without link protein; however, they tend to be less stable, shorter, and to have more irregular spacing between subunits bound to the hyaluronic acid filament.

Articular cartilage is not a homogeneous material. Significant biochemical and morphologic changes occur as the depth increases from the articular surface. With increasing depth, water content decreases, as indicated in Slide III,11. Slide III,12 shows that the collagen content also decreases with increasing depth from the surface, whereas proteoglycan content increases.

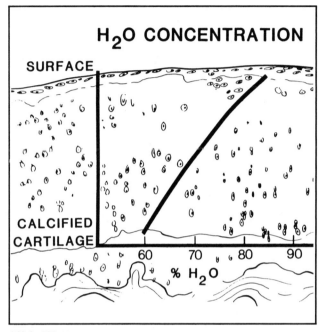

Slide III,11

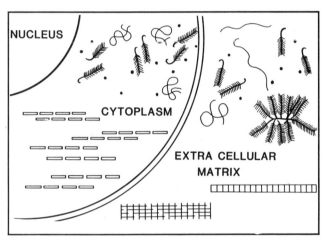

Slide III,10

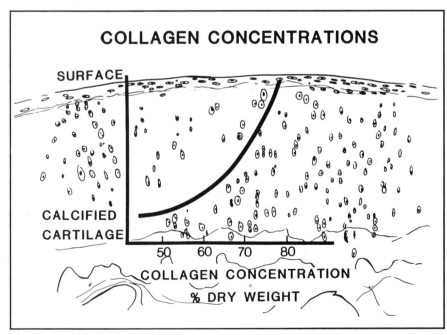

Slide III,12

Repair of Articular Cartilage

Injuries to cartilage can be divided into those that initially degrade the macromolecular organization of the matrix and those that result from direct mechanical injury. Matrix degradation is initiated by breakdown of the proteoglycan molecules, which are subsequently lost from the matrix. Initially, chondrocytes can restore lost proteoglycan, but if the rate of loss exceeds their ability to synthesize new matrix molecules, the damage becomes irreversible. Immobilization of joints causes loss of cartilage proteoglycan. If joint motion is restored, proteoglycan content returns to normal. In infectious arthritis, the initial insult to the cartilage appears to be degradation of proteoglycans. If the infectious process is arrested early, the articular cartilage can be restored to normal. Mechanical injuries, either blunt or penetrating, disrupt the organization of the matrix so severely that the cells cannot restore it.

The Response of Articular Cartilage to Injury and Immobilization

The rabbit articular cartilage in Slide III,13 is stained with safranin-O, which demonstrates the presence of proteoglycans by its red-orange color. In this sample, multiple lacerations were made in the articular surface. One year following injury, there has been no significant repair of these lacerations. The initial response of the chondrocytes to this type of injury is increased matrix synthesis and a limited degree of proliferation, as indicated by the deeper red staining of the matrix. These responses are inadequate to repair the matrix defects, but the defects do not appear to progress to more serious disease.

Slide III,14 illustrates a full-thickness defect through articular cartilage into subchondral bone. Unlike the response shown in Slide III,13, a fibrin clot has formed in the defect because penetration of subchondral bone initiates a vascular response to injury. Even at this stage several days after injury, an active repair process is proceeding.

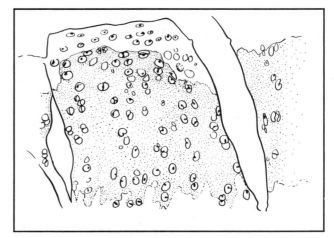

Slide III,13

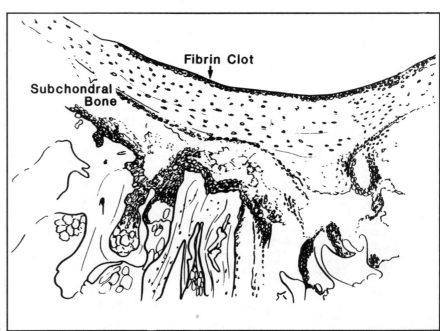

Slide III,14

Slide III,15 shows a two-month followup of the injury shown in Slide III,14. A new articular cartilage matrix has appeared and it stains well for proteoglycans. Cells initially produce a new matrix that appears morphologically and histochemically to resemble the original matrix.

Unfortunately, as noted in Slide III,16 one year after injury, this articular matrix has lost its proteoglycan content and has deteriorated, which is the common result of full-thickness articular cartilage injury. The deterioration of repair cartilage may be related to the inability of the cells to synthesize and organize the organic macromolecular framework of articular cartilage once this framework has been disrupted. With time, this repair matrix becomes increasingly fibrotic and begins to fibrillate; it may eventually leave exposed bone. Current research, including studies of continuous passive motion, reflects attempts to facilitate restoration of a more normal articular cartilage matrix.

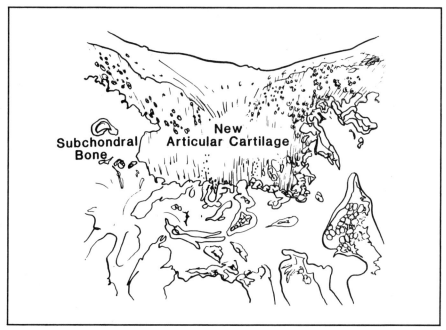

Slide III,15

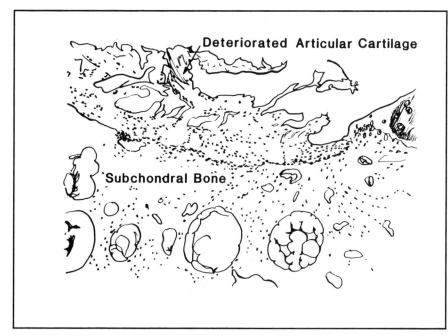

Slide III,16

Slide III,17 is a photomicrograph of the surface contact area of a rigidly immobilized joint. This type of immobilization for a period of weeks produces temporary loss of proteoglycans. The slide demonstrates a loss of staining intensity in the articular cartilage reflecting a loss of proteoglycan aggregates, together with a loss of cartilage thickness. The separation of the cartilage layers is fixation artifact. Prolonged immobilization causes irreversible damage. In contact areas, the severity of changes depends upon the degree of compression. The process is similar to the development of a pressure ulcer of the skin. Here, of course, in cartilage there is no tissue vascularity and different mechanisms are undoubtedly at play. All degrees of severity are observed, beginning with a minimum loss of staining of the matrix at one extreme to full-thickness ulceration of matrix down to subchondral bone at the other extreme. This combination of immobilization and contact area compression is potentially devastating.

Slide III,18 illustrates that changes also occur in the non-contact areas of articular cartilage. Fibrofatty connective tissue proliferation fills the synovial recesses and covers the noncontacting areas of articular cartilage. The process begins at the periphery near the synovial reflection and progresses centripetally. The overgrown cartilage becomes thin, and the tangential layer of cartilage cells is lost. Fibrillation and loss of matrix-staining characteristics soon follow.

Immobilization also causes changes in the joint's other tissues. Slide III,19 shows the disorganization that occurs in an anterior cruciate ligament of an immobilized joint (right) compared to the control (left). Loss of the parallel arrays and disorganization of the immobilized tissue are striking. If joint mobility can be resumed relatively early in the course of a treatment program, the maturation process of the proliferative tissue can be arrested and adhesions can be avoided.

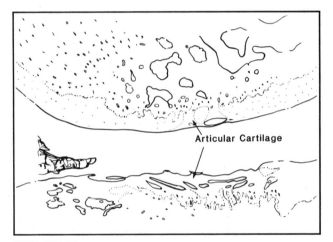

Articular Cartilage

Slide III,17

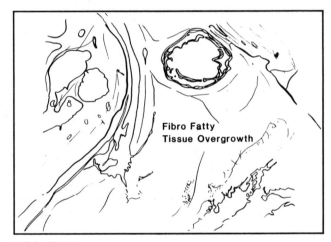

Fibro Fatty Tissue Overgrowth

Slide III,18

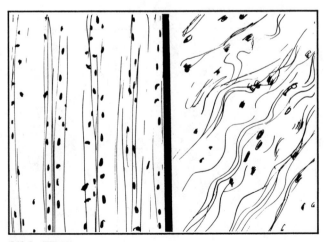

Slide III,19

Osteoarthritis

Osteoarthritis is one of the most common disabling musculoskeletal diseases, yet it remains poorly understood. The early stages of osteoarthritis are particularly unclear since most of the tissue studied comes from patients with advanced disease, as shown in Slide III,20, a radiograph of a severely arthritic knee. The knee has marked loss of cartilage in the medial compartment and osteophyte formation.

The first detectable cartilage changes in osteoarthritis are increased water content, increased glycosaminoglycan content, and increased cell proliferation followed by a gradual decline and disruption of the matrix collagen fibrillar network. Fibrillation and fissuring of the articular cartilage clearly demonstrate the disruption of the matrix caused by the above changes, as shown in the photomicrograph on Slide III,21.

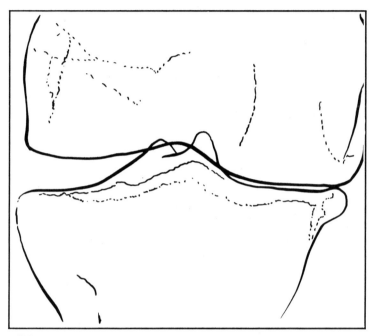

Slide III,20

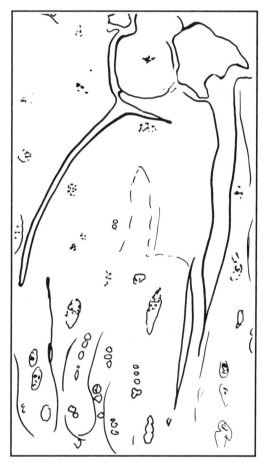

Slide III,21

Cartilage Allografts

Some research centers are using allografts to replace severely damaged articular surfaces. Promising early results have been reported, but the long-term function of these grafts remains unknown. Slide III,22 shows a radiograph of a knee in a patient with severe posttraumatic arthritis. A cartilage allograph has been done on the lateral side. Slide III,23 shows the knee one year after allograft replacement. There is good maintenance of the joint space and no significant collapse or fragmentation of graft.

Tendon

Tendons are dense, regularly arranged connective tissue composed of fibroblasts, collagen, and proteoglycans.

The fibroblasts are responsible for the synthesis of the matrix: collagen and proteoglycans. The major constituent of tendon is type I collagen. Collagen bundles combine to form ordered units of microfibrils, subfibrils, fibrils, and fascicles, which are arranged in closely packed parallel bundles oriented in a distinct longitudinal pattern. This arrangement offers the greatest resistance to tensile (pulling) forces. The fascicles within the tendon are bound together by loose connective tissue termed the endotenon, which permits longitudinal movement of the collagen bundles, as well as providing support to the blood vessels, lymphatics, and nerves.

Tendons that are not enclosed within a sheath and move in a straight direction are surrounded by a loose areolar connective tissue called the paratenon. Tendons that bend sharply, such as the flexor tendons of the hand, are enclosed by a tendon sheath to prevent bow-stringing of the tendon.

Slide III,22

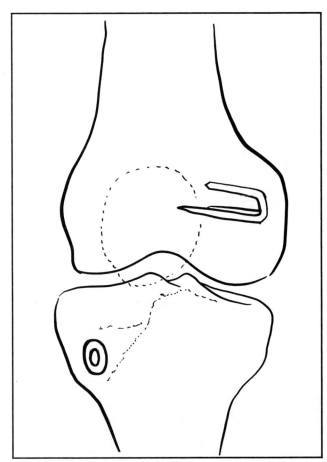

Slide III,23

Tendon Repair

Slide III,24 shows the early repair response at the end of a transected tendon. After the paratenon and tendon are completely cut, the wound fills with inflammatory products (blood cells, nuclear debris and fibrin). This tissue has no tensile strength. During the first week, the union of the tendon stumps is effected by proliferating tissue from the paratenon. Paratenon tissue penetrates the gap and then fills it with undifferentiated and disorganized fibroblasts containing well-developed endoplasmic reticulum. Capillary buds invade the area and together with the fibroblasts create the granulation tissue between the tendon ends seen in Slide III,25.

In the presence of the paratenon and the invading granulation tissue, the fibroblasts begin to take part in the synthesis of collagen as early as the third day. This process begins with an increased concentration of the glycoproteins observed outside the cell. These glycoproteins aid in the polymerization process of the monomeric collagen particles (tropocollagen) that are produced by the fibroblasts. The endoplasmic reticulum of the fibroblasts synthesizes a precursor of collagen that is approximately 2800 nm long and 14 nm wide, with a molecular weight of 340,000 daltons. This triple-chain helix depends upon heat-sensitive hydrogen-bond crosslinks to connect its hydroxyl groups of hydroxyproline to the ketoamide groups of other helices. The critical step in the production of this monomeric collagen (tropocollagen) is the hydroxylation of the proline-rich polypeptide precursors. In the proper milieu, the tropocollagen begins to polymerize into fibrils. These fibrils progressively accumulate more collagen molecules until they have increased in size to become histologically visible as thin wavy forms. The orientation of the collagen fibers between the tendon stumps is perpendicular to the long axis of the tendon. Repair is an active process, and by 10 days following injury the collagen production in the wound has been shown to increase to 15 times that of normal tendons, peaking to 22 times normal levels at 14 to 28 days. The decline in active collagen production is slow, with the level at 84 days still at 15 times normal collagen production. Immunofluorescent studies show that the collagen produced is type I.

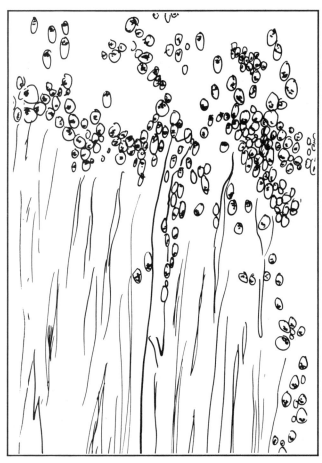

Slide III,24

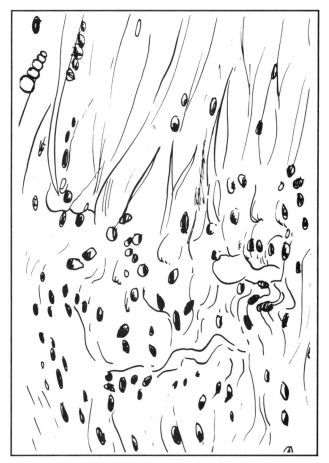

Slide III,25

Slide III,26 shows histologically that during fibroblastic and vascular proliferation the tendon stumps markedly increase in size. Fibroblasts with many collagen fibers bridge the gap and physically unite the tendon ends. The fibrovascular tissue migrating from the paratendinous tissue blends in with the "epitenon" to form the tendon callus.

Slide III,27 shows that during the third and fourth weeks the fibroblasts and collagen fibers near the tendon begin to orient parallel to the long axis of the tendon. The parallel orientation of the new scar tissue is caused by the directional stress placed on the tissue. This stress affects only the collagen near the tendon, while the more peripheral scar tissue remains unorganized. This difference in orientation of collagen fibers in the newly synthesized scar tissue is defined as secondary remodeling. Once again, form reflects function.

The two important activities of secondary remodeling are the increase in tensile strength and the reduction in the mass of scar tissue, both of which continue for many months. Evidence for this activity is seen in that depolymerized collagen can be found even as maturation continues. This depolymerized collagen is in the process of reverting through the monomeric soluble phase, thus reducing the size of the scar. In addition, even though the total collagen mass begins to diminish, tensile strength increases and is related to the remodeling in progress. This increase in tensile strength of the scar suggests a high degree of organization along the lines of stress. Research has documented that a direct proportional increase in production of monomeric collagen is due to an increase in longitudinal tension. This stress also strengthens and increases the bonds between the collagen fibers. These studies also report that a decrease in longitudinal stress results in a decrease in collagen production—a phenomenon that also applies to skin, bone and other connective tissues.

As healing proceeds, collagenization continues; by the 20th week there is only a minimal histologic difference between the scar and the normal tendon. This difference represents a slight increase in vascularity and cellularity.

The healing process of a tendon enclosed by a sheath has been a controversial topic for many years. Early investigation suggested that healing of these tendons was effected by granulation from the tendon sheath, supporting the "one wound-one scar" concept. Some investigators demonstrated that surgically transected digital flexor tendons in the dog healed by a scar produced by fibroblasts derived from the tendon sheath and surrounding tissues. The tendon cells seemed to play no active role in this repair. In other studies, under specially controlled laboratory conditions, investigators have shown healing of partially incised tendons by the tenoblast without assistance from the surrounding tissue cells.

Over the past two decades, several points have been established by tendon-healing research: 1) All tendons have a vascular supply. In sheathed tendons (e.g. flexor tendons of the hand), there is also nourishment by synovial fluid diffusion. 2) Experimentally, tendon cells are capable of proliferating, producing collagen, and reconstructing their own gliding surface in the absence of adhesion ingrowth (granulation reaction). 3) The key to a successful outcome following flexor tendon repair is meticulous restoration of tendon continuity and early passive mobilization. Early mobilization of the tendon reduces adhesions from extrinsic repair, improves collagen alignment along lines of stress and should stimulate intrinsic repair.

Slide III,26

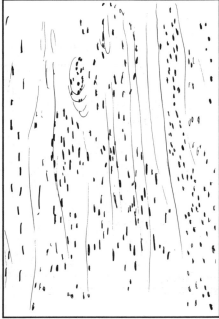

Slide III,27

Intervertebral Disc

Slide III,28, diagrams a lateral view of the spine. Normal motion and stability of the spine depend to a large extent on the intervertebral disc. In young people, the nucleus pulposus and anulus fibrosus can be easily identified, as shown in the schematic diagram. The mechanical properties of the disc are dependent on the organization of the disc components, and on the specific properties of the extracellular matrix. The nucleus can be considered a hydrated gel enclosed by the annular lamina, giving the disc hydrostatic properties. The arrangement of the collagenous lamina allows for disc extensibility. The unit permits distribution of axial loads between the vertebral endplate and the lamina, as illustrated by the lower disc shown in Slide III,28. The properties of tensil strength are attributed to the collagen, whereas compressibility is governed by the proteoglycans of the gel. This arrangement is analogous to articular cartilage, in which the mechanical properties are produced by these same matrix components. The disc, in a sense, has segregated these components more than has articular cartilage.

As shown in Slide III,29, the composition of the disc changes between the nucleus pulposus and the anulus fibrosus and between the inner layers of the anulus and its outer layers. The nucleus has high glycosaminoglycan content with a relatively low collagen content, while the outermost layer of the anulus fibrosus contains mostly collagen with little glycosaminoglycan.

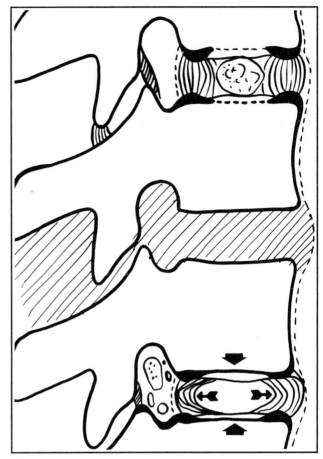

Slide III,28

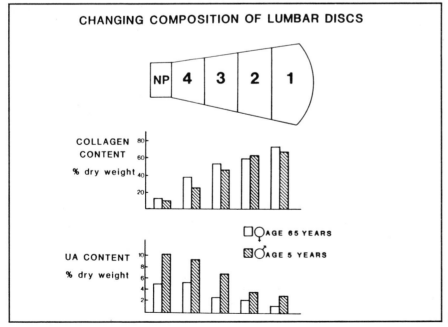

Slide III,29

Age changes the composition of the disc. The young nucleus contains about 85% water and the young anulus contains about 78% water. With age the water content of both disc components falls to about 70%, and disc proteoglycan content decreases while the noncollagen protein content increases.

As illustrated in Slide III,30, disc proteoglycans differ from those of cartilage. The molecules of a disc are smaller and contain relatively more keratan sulfate and protein. In addition, proteoglycan aggregates from a disc are smaller than aggregates from cartilage. Type II collagen forms the fibrillar macromolecular framework of the nucleus pulposus. As noted in Slide III,31, the anulus contains both type I and type II collagen, but the proportion of type I progressively increases from the inner to the outer anulus.

Degenerative changes in the intervertebral disc are defined morphologically in Slide III,32, representing the degenerative disc from a 55-year-old person. More advanced degenerative changes are seen in Slide III,33, a gross specimen of a 75-year-old disc. The anulus border is obscured, distinct structure is lost, the nucleus is fibrosed, the endplate is thinned, the peripheral border bulges, and clefts and fissures are present. These changes are age-related.

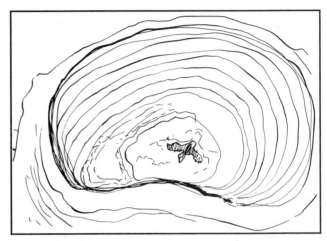

Slide III,32

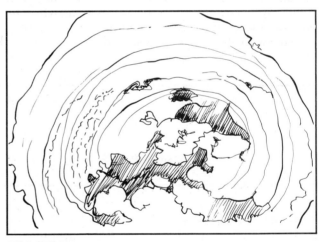

Slide III,33

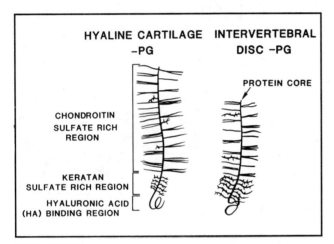

Slide III,30

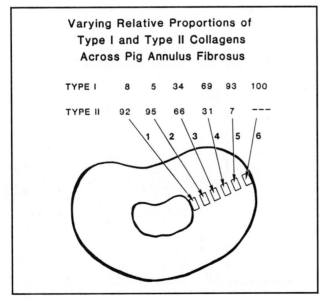

Slide III,31

Some Generalized Disorders of Connective Tissue

Synthesis and assembly of connective-tissue matrix macromolecules follows a precisely ordered sequence of steps. Abnormalities in any of these steps can cause significant disturbances of connective-tissue function. To demonstrate, three genetically determined disorders of connective tissue will be discussed: osteogenesis imperfecta; Ehlers-Danlos syndrome; and Marfan's syndrome.

Osteogenesis Imperfecta

Osteogenesis imperfecta classically has been considered a bone disorder. Recent studies, however, demonstrate specific defects of collagen in tissues from patients with osteogenesis imperfecta. These include increased synthesis of type III collagen and decreased synthesis of type I collagen. Alterations in collagen hydroxylation and possible abnormalities of collagen crosslinking have also been reported.

There are two varieties of osteogenesis imperfecta: osteogenesis imperfecta congenita and osteogenesis imperfecta tarda. Osteogenesis imperfecta congenita is characterized by severe involvement. At birth there are numerous fractures and the child is often born dead or survives only a brief time. Osteogenesis imperfecta is usually inherited as an autosomal dominant disorder. There are a few well-documented cases for recessive inheritance in the congenita form. Histologically there is a marked decrease in bone and a lack of maturation. Slide III,34 shows fractures of all long bones in both the upper and lower extremities in a child with osteogenesis imperfecta congenita.

Osteogenesis imperfecta tarda has a variable course. As shown in Slide III,35, in some cases a serpentine-shaped fibula results from repeated fractures. In more severe cases a saber shin has been noted. At times, even without evidence of fracture or deformity, there may be severe osteopenia. In some severe cases multiple roddings of the long bones can be helpful in preventing fractures and severe deformity. Osteogenesis imperfecta in tissue other than bone can be seen in blue sclera, and as shown in Slide III,36 a whiter area adjacent to the cornea. It should be noted that blue sclera are not infrequently seen in persons free of disease and are occasionally absent in patients with disease. In osteogenesis imperfecta, the skin is characteristically thin and translucent. Osteosclerosis has been associated with deafness. The teeth often have an amber yellowish brown or translucent bluish gray coloration, which has been termed dentinogenesis imperfecta. Root canals and pulp chambers tend to become obliterated.

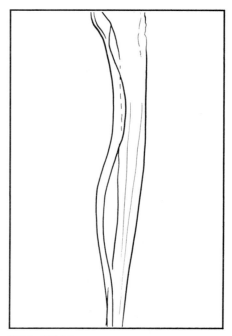

Slide III,35

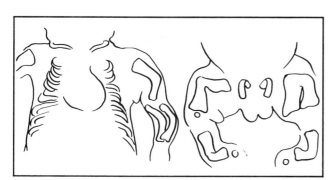

Slide III,34

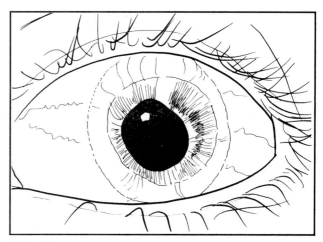

Slide III,36

Ehlers-Danlos Syndrome

Ehlers-Danlos syndrome is characterized by hyperextensible skin, (Slide III,37) hypermobile joints (Slide III,38), fragile tissues including blood vessels, and a bleeding diathesis. Recently, this syndrome has been reclassified with particular emphasis on biochemical defects. Types I, II, and III show an autosomal dominant pattern of inheritance. Type I, the gravis type, is characterized by marked skin hyperextensibility, joint hypermobility, skin fragility, moderate bruising, associated musculoskeletal deformity, varicose veins, and premature delivery of pregnancy due to ruptured membranes. Type II, the mitis type, is a milder form of type I. Type III is characterized by joint hypermobility and musculoskeletal deformities.

Type IV, or the ecchymotic type, is inherited in a dominant manner, although recently an example of autosomal recessive inheritance has been noted. Type IV is characterized by marked skin fragility, bruising, arterial ruptures, and bowel perforations. Fibroblasts from patients with type IV disorder synthesize type I collagen, but do not synthesize the type III collagen normally found in arterial walls and the gastrointestinal system. The lack of this type III collagen in the arterial walls and bowel predisposes them to rupture.

Type V Ehlers-Danlos syndrome is characterized by marked skin hyperextensibility and some joint hypermobility. Biochemical studies in fibroblast cultures show a decrease in lysl oxidase activity necessary for collagen crosslinking, and the fibroblasts synthesize excessively soluble collagen. Individuals with type V Ehlers-Danlos excrete large amounts of hydroxylysine glycosides and L-valyl proline, which are degradation products of collagen and elastin. These data suggest impaired collagen crosslinking so necessary for stabilization and strength of the collagen fibers.

Type VI Ehlers-Danlos syndrome, or the ocular type, is characterized by marked skin hyperextensibility and joint hypermobility. Type VI is frequently complicated by fragility of the cornea and sclera, as well as scoliosis. A recessive disorder, type VI is characterized by a marked reduction in the hydroxylysine content of collagen and a specific deficiency in collagen lysl hydroxylase. These biochemical aberrations lead to a deficiency in intermolecular crosslinks.

Type VII Ehlers-Danlos syndrome is similar to dermatosparaxis described in cows and sheep. Patients with this disorder are of short stature, have stretchable velvety skin, hyperextensible joints, and multiple joint dislocations. Inheritance is autosomal recessive. Biochemically, these individuals are deficient in procollagen peptidase, the enzyme which cleaves the amino terminal extension of the collagen molecule. Clinical signs are due to impairment of aggregation and collagen crosslinking because of the presence of the amino terminal extensions.

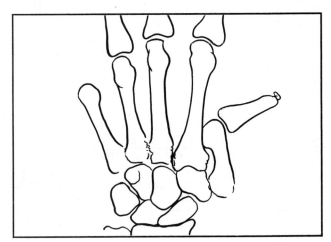

Slide III,37

Slide III,38

Marfan's Syndrome

Marfan's syndrome is an autosomal dominant disorder that occurs with approximately the same frequency as osteogenesis imperfecta. The biochemical defect in Marfan's syndrome may be due to a deficit in collagen synthesis or fibril assembly. Marfan's syndrome is characterized by excessive limb length, scoliosis, chestwall deformity and joint laxity. Ectopic lentis, myopia and retinal detachment are observed in the eye. Death is frequently caused by a dissecting aortic aneurysm, although mitral valve disease also occurs. Slide III,39 shows a radiograph demonstrating the long thin fingers and the flexion deformity of the little finger characteristic of Marfan's syndrome.

A frequent complication of Marfan's syndrome is scoliosis, which can be severe as noted in Slide III,40. The ectopic lens is seen in Slide III,41. More than 70% of patients with Marfan's syndrome will show some abnormality of the lens on careful examination.

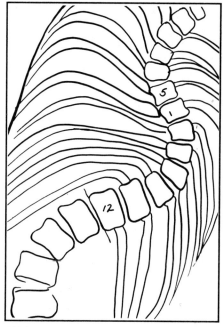

Slide III,40

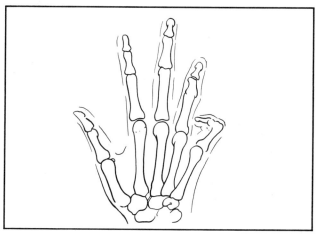

Slide III,39

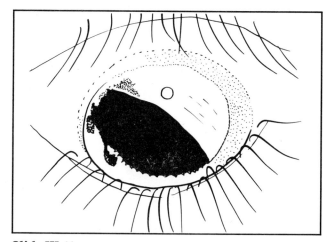

Slide III,41

Neuromuscular Disorders

Understanding the differential diagnosis of neuromuscular disorders requires a knowledge of the elements of the lower motor neuron and the disease processes that can affect each of these elements. These elements include the anterior horn cell, the peripheral nerve fiber, the neuromuscular junction, and the striated muscle fiber.

In neuropathies, muscle changes are a secondary response to the primary disease and consist of the following abnormalities: small angular fibers; target fibers; group atrophy (types I and II fibers); and fiber type grouping.

Slide III,42 is an illustration of group muscle atrophy. The left-hand portion of the slide shows that all the muscle fibers of both fiber types, the darker type I and the lighter type II, are atrophied. The atrophy is geographical or regional and adjacent muscle fiber groups, as shown in the lower right-hand corner of the slide, may remain unaffected by the disease. The muscle fibers on the lower right-hand side of the slide are plump and appear healthy. When regional atrophy of whole groups of muscle fibers

occurs, regardless of the fiber types contained within the group, this form of atrophy is referred to as group atrophy. The reason both muscle types are affected in group atrophy is that each neuromuscular junction innervates an entire region of muscle fibers. Each region contains both types of muscle fibers; therefore, both fiber types atrophy. Group muscle atrophy is a hallmark of lower motor neuron disease and may be seen in such disorders as spinal muscle atrophy, Kugelberg-Welander's disease, and poliomyelitis.

Slide III,43 shows a photomicrograph of skeletal muscle in cross-section stained with a histochemical preparation. Type I fibers are darkly stained and type II fibers are lightly stained. Normally, the darkly stained fibers should outnumber the lightly stained fibers by a 3:2 ratio. The loss of a specific fiber type, as shown in this slide, is termed fiber-type grouping and is characteristic of a primary myopathy. In this slide, the large pattern of homogeneous fibers is well demonstrated. It should be emphasized that atrophy caused by degenerative conditions should always involve both fiber types in contrast to disuse atrophy, which involves only type-II fibers.

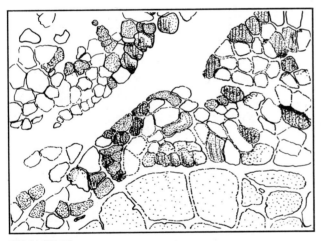

Slide III,42

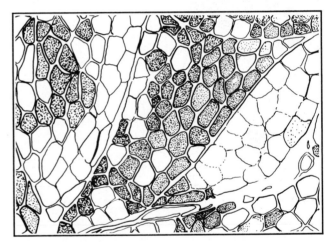

Slide III,43

Primary Disorders of Muscle

Muscular dystrophy (pseudohypertrophies, progressive, X-linked recessive dystrophy) represents the most common clinical muscular disorder in children. The incidence of this disease is approximately 20 to 30 per 100,000 live male births. The prevalence is 3 per 100,000.

Classically, pseudohypertrophic (Duchenne's) muscular dystrophy affects only males who have inherited the condition from their carrier mothers. A high mutation rate exists, with up to one-third of cases representing mutations. How the genetic disorder affects the form and function of the muscle is not known. Duchenne's muscular dystrophy typically presents at 3 to 5 years of age with signs of proximal muscle weakness, such as a waddling gait. Up to one-third of patients are mildly mentally retarded. At 11 to 13 years of age, the child loses the ability to walk unaided. Death usually occurs in the early twenties from cardiomyopathy, or earlier from pulmonary insufficiency. Creatine phosphokinase (CPK) elevation, and positive findings on electromyograph and muscle biopsy confirm the diagnosis. Slide III,44 is a histologic section illustrating an advanced state of this disease. There is a marked increase in the variability of muscle fiber diameters with proliferation of endomysial and perimysial connective tissue and fat; muscle fiber necrosis is extensive.

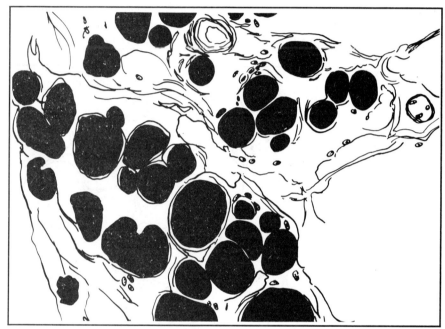

Slide III,44

The inflammatory myopathies dermatomyositis and poliomyelitis are acquired disorders of muscle seen at any age. The two disorders are similar except that dermatomyositis is frequently seen in childhood and in late adult years and affects skin, whereas poliomyelitis may occur at any age and is usually not associated with other connective tissue diseases. In both, muscle weakness occurs in a proximal symmetrical distribution. This pattern is in contrast to the asymmetrical pattern of proximal involvement in the dystrophic muscle diseases. The course of dermatomyositis is variable and spontaneous remissions in childhood can occur. The disease may be associated with occult malignancies in nearly 20% of the cases.

Slides III,45 and III,46 illustrate the histologic features common to both disorders. In Slide III,45 atrophic fibers with scattered necrosis and collections of inflammatory cells are noted. Unlike other muscle diseases, there is no hypertrophy of muscle fibers (Slide III,46). Inflammatory changes are present in a perivascular location. This finding is present in only 60% to 70% of cases. In childhood dermatomyositis, *perifascicular atrophy* is most commonly seen, and may be secondary to vascular involvement, with ischemia of the small endarterioles of the muscle fascicle.

Slide III,45

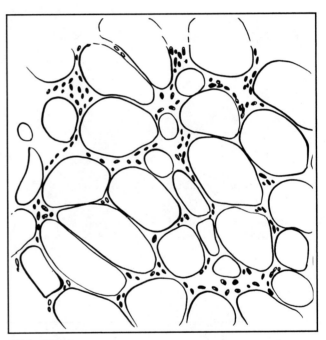

Slide III,46

Muscle Damage Secondary to Circulatory Compromise

A compartment syndrome is a condition in which increased pressure within a limited space compromises the circulation and results in necrosis of the contents of that space. The earliest finding and *sine qua non* of an acute compartment syndrome is increased pressure. A prerequisite for the development of increased tissue pressure is an envelope restricting the volume available to the enclosed tissue. Such envelopes include the epimysium, fascia, the skin, casts, or other circumferential dressings. A compartment syndrome usually does not develop immediately after injury. The syndrome will not occur until the pressure in the compartment rises above capillary levels, as shown in Slide III,47. In the usual case, the lag phase from time of injury to the development of a compartment syndrome averages six to eight hours, but the lag phase may be as long as two days.

Measurement of compartment pressure, as illustrated in Slide III,48, will allow early diagnosis and treatment of compartment syndromes. The compartments requiring decompression pressures in normotensive patients vary and are related to the patient's diastolic pressures. Compartment pressures approaching the patient's diastolic pressures are strongly suspect, but should be complemented with the clinical examination of the patient.

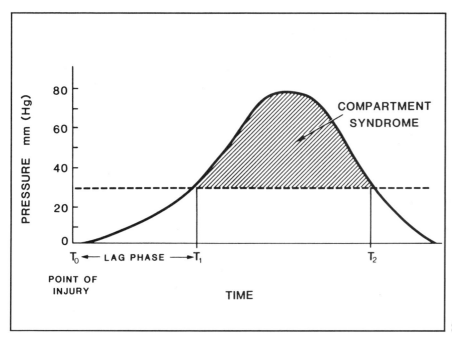

Slide III,47

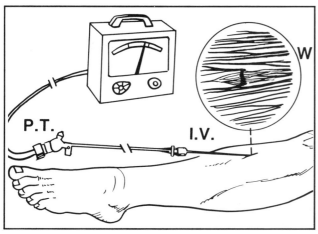

Slide III,48

Nerve Degeneration and Regeneration

Nerve Degeneration

Nerve injuries are classified into three types: The first type is neurotmesis, a complete severance of a nerve. The second type is axonotmesis, usually a crushing injury to a nerve that breaks axons in the myelin sheaths. The epineurium, endoneurium, and perineurium are usually intact. Wallerian degeneration occurs distally. The third type is neurapraxia, which is a compression injury. Motor paralysis is usually present, but there may be only partial sensory loss. Wallerian degeneration is not common with this type of injury.

Denervation can be complete or partial. Complete denervation is caused by axonotmesis or neurotmesis. There is no conduction distally after wallerian degeneration progresses. In partial lesions, conduction continues to occur across the lesion, but the evoked response is abnormal and strength-duration curves are shifted to the right.

After a nerve has been lacerated, the two stumps separate, and the gap fills with clot. There is marked proximal swelling with intra-and extracellular edema lasting approximately one week. Metabolism of the Schwann cells and the epineurial cells is increased, and retrograde degeneration occurs. In cutting injuries, this retrograde degeneration is slight, but in blast or crush injuries it may be 1 to 3 centimeters in extent. Conduction velocity is reduced. With an axonal injury, the events occurring proximally include chromatolysis, with nuclear eccentricity and nuclear enlargement. The nerve cell swells. There is disappearance of granules (Nissl bodies) and increased RNA synthesis. Also glucose-6-phosphodehydrogenase (G6PD) production increases, with an increase in the glucose metabolism via the anaerobic pentose pathway. Lipid synthesis is increased.

Distally, a process called "wallerian degeneration" occurs in which all neural elements distal to the injury site die. (Wallerian degeneration does *not* refer to any changes in the proximal stump.) Additional changes include an increase in production of digestive enzymes with the neuronal elements breaking down within a week. The myelin becomes fragmented and digested by the Schwann cells, a process usually completed in 6 weeks. The nerve shrinks, the endoneurial sheaths decrease in size or disappear completely, and conductivity is lost after three or four days. This process is illustrated in Slides III,49 and III,50.

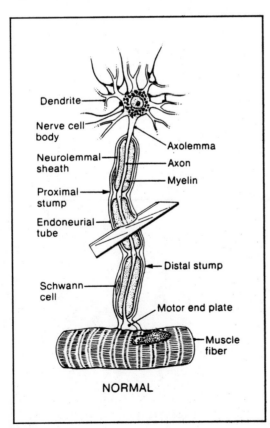

Slide III,49

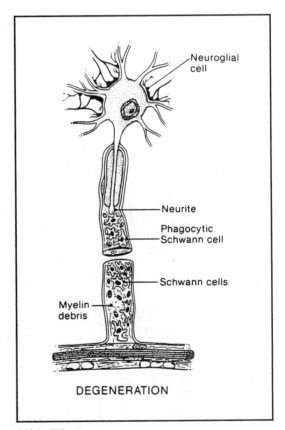

Slide III,50

As shown in Slide III,51, if nerve continuity is not restored, the result is a large bulbous prominence at the end of the proximal nerve stump called a neuroma. The enlargement of the distal stump at the area of the laceration is called a glioma.

Nerve Regeneration

Two to three days after laceration, nerve regeneration begins with the proliferation of all cellular elements in the proximal and distal stumps. After one week, Schwann cells become most active, and there is orientation of the mesenchymal cells after debridement of necrotic material has occurred.

In the distal stump there is a longitudinal proliferation of the fibroblasts proximally, and a proliferation of the Schwann cells. The epineurium, endoneurium and perineurium participate in this healing process, attempting to form a bridge across the gap site. When this process fails, a glioma results. After successful repair, with penetration of new axons a proper orientation of Schwann cells begin forming a fresh myelin layer. During the next 1 to 3 weeks there is an anabolic trophic phase in the proximal stump of the cell body. Simultaneously, the axons begin to regenerate and sprout. Regenerating axons require restoration of lipids and proteins, made in the cell body and transmitted through the nerve to the area of

regeneration. Neuronal elongation distally originates at growth cones. These growth cones are a profuse elaboration of microspikes that explore an area and determine direction of regrowth. There appears to be some biological signal for this nerve sprouting. Trophic interactions have been demonstrated by a tissue substance that stimulates this sprouting. As these new axons penetrate the distal nerve segment, Schwann cells begin to produce myelin. This remyelinization process, however, never achieves the normal state. The regenerated nerve has a smaller perineurium, smaller myelin sheaths, and smaller endoneurial tubes. Conduction times are usually diminished. This regeneration process is illustrated in Slide III,52.

Regeneration has been studied in the laboratory clinically by the following methods: functional; biochemical; anatomical; axonal transport; electrophysiological. Functional methods include walking patterns, use of the hand in time-motion studies, withdrawal-to-pain stimulus, muscle mass/strength and contraction. Biochemical methods include collagen and myelin assays. Anatomical methods include the histology of end organs, muscle sections, and nerve fiber counts. Axonal transport includes use of radioactive labels or horseradish peroxidase as markers to monitor the transport of these substances through the regenerating nerve tissue. Electrophysiological methods commonly used to determine regeneration of nerves include nerve conduction velocity, axon potential, and electromyograms.

REGENERATION WITHOUT SUTURE

Slide III,51

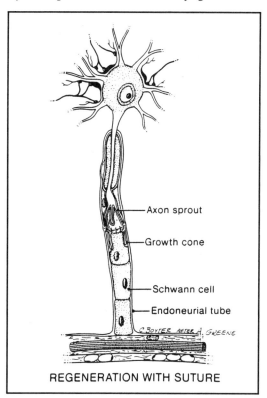

— Axon sprout

— Growth cone

— Schwann cell

— Endoneurial tube

REGENERATION WITH SUTURE

Slide III,52

Wound Repair

The repair of damaged tissue requires the concerted action of many specialized cell types, including leukocytes, connective tissue cells, and endothelial cells. These cells invade the wound area in a precise sequence that may be important for the proper maturation and restoration of the traumatized tissue. It appears there are specific chemical factors regulating both the migration and proliferation of the cells involved in wound repair. The levels of these chemotactic factors and mitogens present at the wound site appear to control, in large part, the order and magnitude of the cellular influxes into the wound area. These early events are probably similar in both soft and hard connective-tissue repair in which the formation of granulation tissue is an intermediate stage. Other factors may direct the differentiation of stem cells in the granulation tissue toward bone, tendon or muscle.

Our understanding of the process of wound repair is incomplete; however, some aspects are known. Slide III,53 illustrates the importance of the initial wound hypoxia in attracting new capillaries into the wound area. A wound chamber with an oxygen-permeable cover (circles) attracts very few capillaries compared to the chamber with an oxygen-impermeable cover (squares). Together with the low oxygen tension in the wound, chemoattractants from the blood clot and resident cells, some of which are listed on Slide III,54, play an important role. Chemoattractants are poorly characterized compounds produced at the wound site to attract reparative cells by a chemical gradient. Not only must cells be attracted to the wound, they must be encouraged to remain, multiply, and produce matrix.

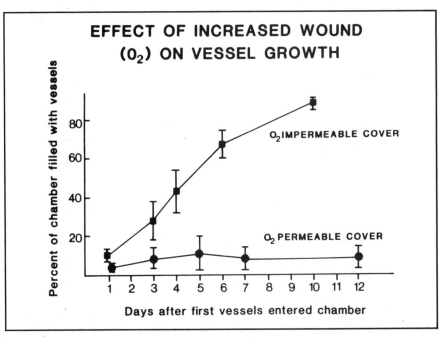

Slide III,53

CHEMOATTRACTANTS IN WOUND REPAIR

CHEMOATTRACTANT	TARGET	RECRUIT
▪C_{5A}, PLATLET FACTOR 4,	▪INFLAMMATORY CELLS	PHAGOCYTES
▪ELASTIN PEPTIES,	NEUTROPHILIS	
▪F-MET PEPTIDES	MONOCYTES	
▪PDGF, FIBRONECTIN,	▪CONNECTIVE TISSUE CELLS	MATRIX PRODUCING CELLS
▪LYMPHOKINES, MONOKINES,	FIBROBLAST	
▪COMPLEMENT PEPTIDES	SMOOTH MUSCLE CELLS	
▪FIBRONECTIN, LAMININ,	▪ENDOTHELIAL CELLS	VASCULAR SYSTEM
▪MONOKINES		

Slide III,54

Chapter 3 • Soft Tissue

Slide III,55 lists several mitogenic and growth factors found at wound sites that are thought to be important in wound healing. (PDGF = platelet-derived growth factor; MDGF = monocyte-derived growth factor; AMDGF = alveolar-macrophage derived growth factor; MDEGF = Macrophage-derived endothelial cell growth factor; ECDGF = endothelial cell-derived growth factor).

Slide III,56 summarizes present thought on soft-tissue wound healing.

GROWTH FACTORS PRESENT DURING WOUND REPAIR

FACTOR	SOURCE	TARGET	APPEARANCE
◗PDGF	–PLATELETS	FIBROBLASTS SMOOTH MUSCLE	WITHIN MINUTES
◗MDGF AMDGF	–MONOCYTES –ALVEOLAR MACROPHAGES	FIBROBLASTS	24–48 HOURS
◗MDECGF	–MACROPHAGES	ENDOTHELIAL CELLS	24–48 HOURS
◗ECDGF	–ENDOTHELIAL CELLS	FIBROBLASTS SMOOTH MUSCLE	5–7 DAYS

Slide III,55

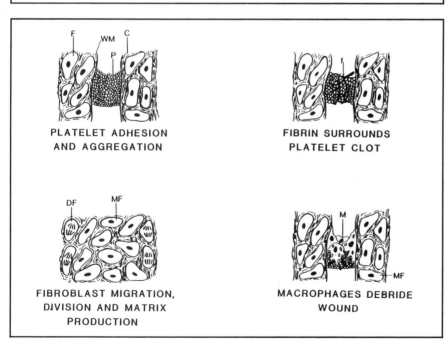

PLATELET ADHESION AND AGGREGATION

FIBRIN SURROUNDS PLATELET CLOT

FIBROBLAST MIGRATION, DIVISION AND MATRIX PRODUCTION

MACROPHAGES DEBRIDE WOUND

Slide III,56

97

Selected Bibliography

Cartilage and Intervertebral Disc

Adams P, Eyre DR, Muir H: Biochemical aspects of development and ageing of human lumbar intervertebral discs. Rheumat and Rehab 1977; 16:22-29.

Buckwalter JA: Proteoglycan structure and calcifying cartilage. Clin Ortho Rel Res 1983; 172:185-210.

Buckwalter JA, Rosenberg LC: Electron microscopic studies of cartilage proteoglycans: Direct evidence for the variable length of the chondroitin sulfate rich region of the proteoglycan subunit core protein. J Biol Chem 1982; 257:9830-9839.

Buckwalter JA, Rosenberg LC, Teng L-H: The effect of link protein on proteoglycan aggregate structure. J Biol Chem 1984; 259:5361-5363.

Buckwalter JA, Pedrini A, Tudisco C, et al: Proteoglycans of human infant intervertebral disc. Electron microscopic and biochemical studies. J Bone and Joint Surg 1985; 67A:284-294.

Buckwalter JA, Kuettner KE, Thonar EJ: Age related changes in articular cartilage proteoglycans: Electron microscopic studies. J Ortho Res 1985; 3:251-257.

Buckwalter JA: Fine structural studies of human intervertebral disc, in White AA, Gordon SL (eds): Proceedings of the Workshop on Idiopathic Low Back Pain, St. Louis, C.V. Mosby, 1982, pp 108-143.

Buckwalter JA: Articular cartilage. Instructional Course Lectures. St Louis, C.V. Mosby, 1984, 33:349-370.

Bushell GR, Ghosh P, Taylor TFK, et al: Proteoglycan chemistry of the intervertebral disks. Clin Orthop 1977; 129:115-123.

Comper W, Laurent R: Physiological Function of Connective Tissue Polysaccharides. Phys Rev 1978; 58:255.

Eyre DR: Collagen: molecular diversity in the body's protein scaffold. Science 1980; 207:1315.

Harris E, Parker H, Radin E, et al: Effects of proteolytic enzymes on structural and mechanical properties of cartilage. Arthritis Rheum 1972; 15:497.

Kempson G: The mechanical properties of articular cartilage, in Sokoloff L (ed): The Joints and Synovial Fluid, II, New York, Academic Press, 1980.

Mankin HJ: The response of articular cartilage to mechanical injury. J Bone and Joint Surg 1982; 64A:460.

Maroudas A: Physicochemical properties of articular cartilage, in Adult Articular Cartilage, ed 2. Turnbridge Wells, Kent. Pitman Medical Publishing Co, Ltd, 1979.

Maroudas A: Physical chemistry of cartilage and intevertebral disc, in Sokoloff L (ed): The Joints and Synovial Fluid, II, New York, Academic Press, 1980.

Stockwell RA, Meachim G: The Chondrocytes, in Freeman MAR (ed):Adult Articular Cartilage, ed 2, Turnbridge Wells, Kent. Pitman Medical Publishing Co, Ltd, 1979.

Neuromuscular Disorders

Brooks MH: A Clinician's View of Neuromuscular Disease. Baltimore, Williams and Wilkins, 1977.

Dubowitz V, Brooks MH: Muscle Biopsy: A Modern Approach. Philadelphia, WB Saunders, 1973.

Matsen FA, Winquist RA, Krugmire RB: Diagnosis and management of compartmental syndromes. J Bone Joint Surg 1980; 62A:286-291.

Mubarak SK, Hargens AR, Owen CA, et al: The wick catheter technique for measurement of intramuscular pressure: A new research and clinical tool. J Bone Joint Surg 1976; 58A:1016-1021.

Whitesides TE, Harada H, Morimotokk: Compartment syndromes and the role of fasciotomy, its parameters and techniques. Instructional Course Lectures. St Louis, C.V. Mosby, 1977, 26:179-196.

Peripheral Nerves

Brunelli G, Monini L, Brunelli F: Problems in nerve lesions surgery. Microsurgery 1985; 6:187-198.

Dyck PJ, Thomas PK, Lambert EH, et al: Peripheral Neuropathy. Philadelphia, WB Saunders, 1984.

Omer GE, Jr: Management of Peripheral Nerve Problems. Philadelphia, WB Saunders, 1980.

Wound Healing

Shoshan S: Wound healing, in International Review of Connective Tissue Research, IX, New York, Academic Press, 1981.

Chapter IV

Pathology

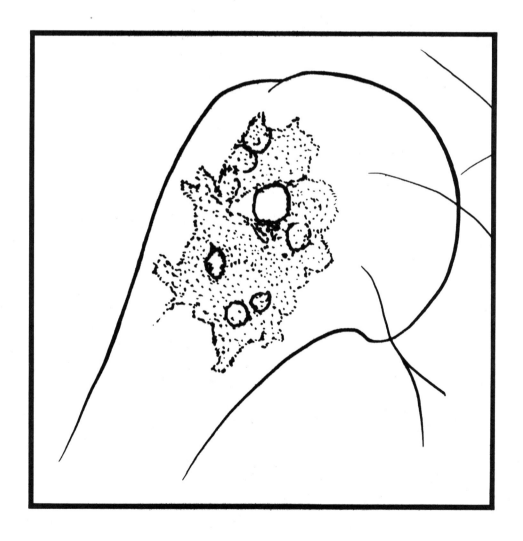

This chapter will discuss musculoskeletal neoplasia, osteomyelitis, synovial disease, and osteonecrosis. It is not intended to be a comprehensive review of these disease processes. The discussion does not include all the important clinical conditions with which the practicing orthopaedist should be familiar, but does illustrate the variable clinical presentations of pathologic conditions and their interpretation. After completing this section, the reader should be able to correlate clinical presentation with pathophysiology and understand the basic pathologic phenomena involved.

Musculoskeletal Neoplasia

Bone Tumors

Primary bone tumors usually arise within the medullary canal, whether they originate from the osteoblastic cell line, chondroblastic cell line, fibroblastic cell line, or marrow cells. The clinical presentation of each of these lesions is dependent upon 1) the growth pattern of the tumor; and 2) the reaction of the host bone to that tumor. As a rule, tumors of different histologic types but with similar growth patterns will present similarly. Tumors of the same histologic type but with different growth patterns will present differently. Because it is the tumor's clinical presentation with which the orthopaedist is confronted, it is axiomatic that a patient must have a thorough history, complete physical examination, and plain radiographs. Once the presenting clinical information is understood, the appropriate management can usually be instituted.

We assume that all tumors arise from a single cell that loses the normal restraints to growth. The two specific defects are lack of contact inhibition and loss of cell cohesiveness. Lack of contact inhibition means that cell division continues despite the crowding of the cells. A simplistic but useful concept is that benign tumors lack contact inhibitors but retain cell cohesiveness, while malignant cells have neither contact inhibition nor cell cohesiveness. The continued growth of the tumor cells is dependent most on the growth pattern of the tumor and not on its specific histology.

Those tumors or non-neoplastic lesions, such as a cyst or a Brodie abscess, that grow slowly enough for the surrounding bone to respond usually present with a well-developed margin of compact bone, sometimes called a "sclerotic margin," completely surrounding the lesions. Slide IV,1 diagrammatically illustrates the radiographic features of this type of lesion. Slide IV,2 shows a radiograph of a non-ossifying fibroma illustrating the least aggressive growth pattern. There is a prominent reactive medullary bone rim or sclerotic margin and an "expanded" but intact cortex. The eccentricity and metaphyseal location of this particular lesion occurring in a young patient are characteristic of a non-ossifying fibroma. Usually during this phase the patient is asymptomatic. As the tumor grows the cortex is invaded and eroded, but the periosteum has time to respond and maintain the cortical bone. This response pattern produces the so-called expanded appearance on the radiograph diagrammed in Slide IV,3. These lesions may exhibit limited growth potential and spontaneously resolve without threatening the integrity of the bone or may significantly weaken the bone and require surgical removal. They are almost always benign and can be observed without biopsy when a pathologic fracture is not a threat.

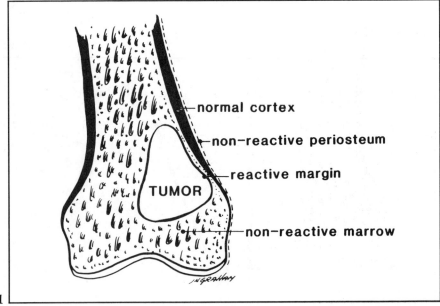

Slide IV,1

100

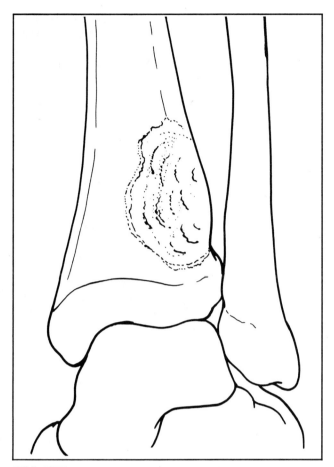

Slide IV,2

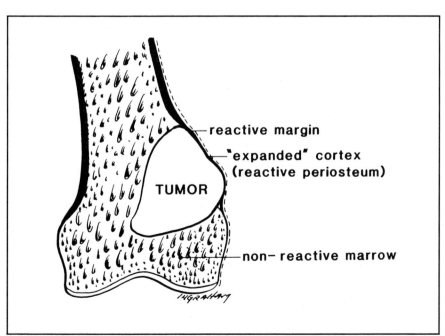

Slide IV,3

Tumors that grow more rapidly may not permit the bone time to respond and will have a less well-developed margin. Slide IV,4 shows a radiograph typifying a more aggressive growth pattern in that there is no reactive medullary rim of bone. Despite destruction of the cortex, the periosteum has maintained its continuity and confined the lesion. These tumors usually grow by pushing their margin into the surrounding bone with minimal invasion between trabeculae. The lesions usually have a minimal medullary border (narrow transition zone). They destroy the cortex completely with minimal periosteal reaction, but do not penetrate the periosteum. Slide IV,5 diagrammatically illustrates the radiographic features of the lesions. These tumors will not spontaneously resolve and must be treated. Slide IV,6 shows a distal tibial lesion with a broad transition zone, absent cortex, and minimal periosteal reaction. The transition zone proximally and distally is narrow, suggesting aggressiveness. Slide IV,7 is a photograph of the gross specimen shown radiographically in Slide IV,6. The matrix is focally calcified, a pattern typical of cartilage. This chondrosarcoma has invaded between preexisting cancellous bone and has replaced the cortex. It is contained by the fibrous periosteum. Slide IV,8 shows a femur with a lesion that has changes illustrative of more aggressive growth. The lesion does not have a well-delineated medullary border, but rather an ill-defined broad transition zone. The cortex is thin and blurred, indicating possible transgression by the tumor.

The lack of a periosteal reaction indicates more rapid growth. The lesion straddles the epiphysis and metaphysis, a finding suggestive of an actively growing tumor. Patients with lesions in this category should be carefully evaluated before surgical intervention.

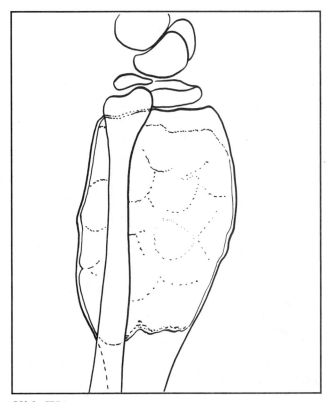

Slide IV,4

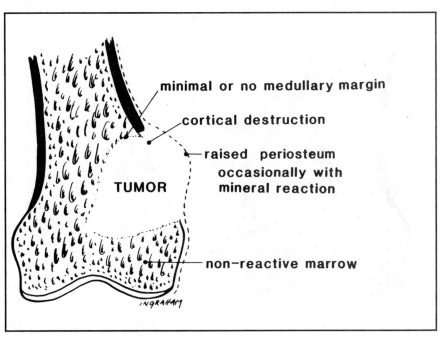

Slide IV,5

minimal or no medullary margin

cortical destruction

raised periosteum occasionally with mineral reaction

TUMOR

non-reactive marrow

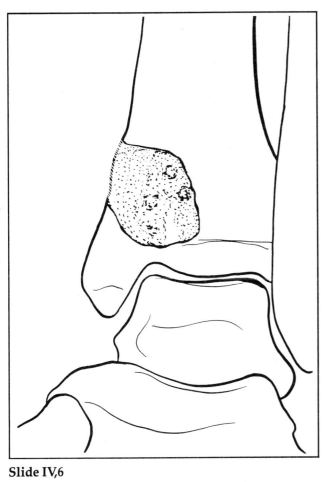

Slide IV,6

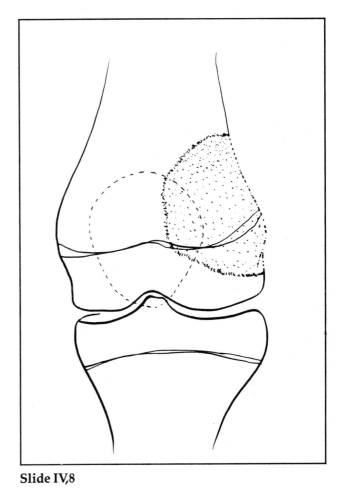

Slide IV,8

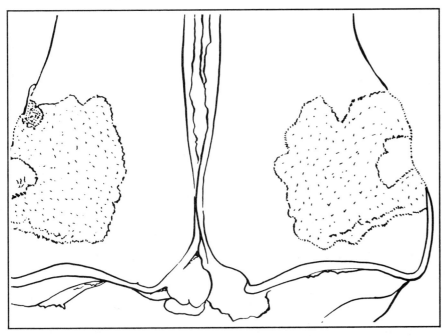

Slide IV,7

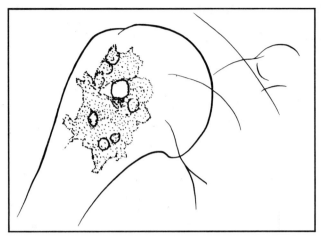

Slide IV,9

The matrix of a lesion may be suggested by its radiographic appearance. Slide IV,9 shows a radiograph of a proximal humerus with regular, diffuse radiodensities in the shape of rings or nodules characteristic of calcified cartilage. The prominence of calcification implies maturation and low biologic aggressiveness. In Slide IV,10, the focal zone of calcification represents a benign cartilage mass; the lytic, poorly defined medullary areas, however, represent an aggressive tumor. The endosteal scalloping of the cortex within the lytic areas confirms the biologic aggressiveness. The combination of an area of calcification and lysis suggests a chondrosarcoma arising in association with a benign endochondroma. Slide IV,11 depicts the gross specimen shown radiographically in Slide IV,10. There is endosteal erosion in the aggressive portion of the tumor. Fluffy densities with a trabecular pattern can usually be recognized as

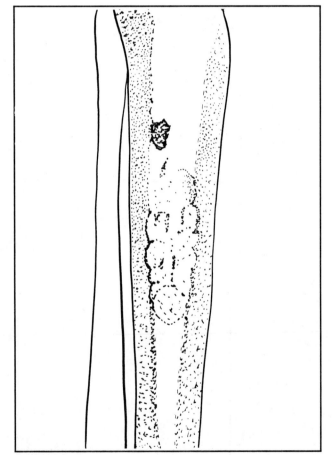

Slide IV,10

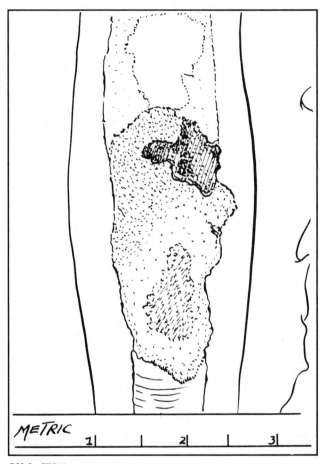

Slide IV,11

bone. Slide IV,12 shows an osteosarcoma in the proximal tibia. The mineralization pattern arranged in spicules is typical of bone. In this case it is produced by the neoplasm. The increased medullary density also represents production of bone by the tumor. The hazy density (often called "ground glass") seen in Slide IV,13 is usually tissue specific for fibrous dysplasia. Slide IV,14 is a photomicrograph of fibrous dysplasia showing the ground glass appearance, which is due to the innumerable mineralized woven bone spicules rather than to the fibrous tissue.

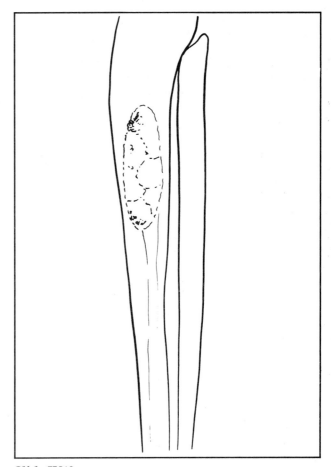

Slide IV,13

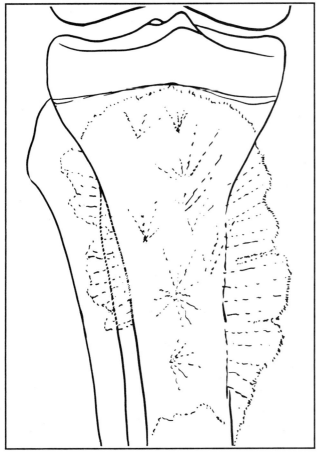

Slide IV,12

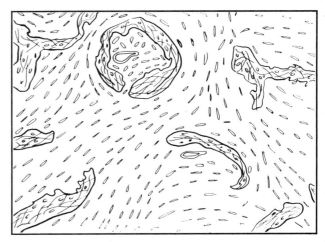

Slide IV,14

The anatomic site within the bone may also provide a significant diagnostic clue. A lesion that presents in the secondary ossification center of a child, as illustrated in Slide IV,15, is a chondroblastoma until proved otherwise. The epiphyseal lesion is well defined with minimal expansion of the cortex and no soft-tissue mass. The lack of matrix is a common finding in chondroblastoma. A lesion involving the epiphysis and metaphysis, immediately adjacent to the subchondral bone in an adult, as illustrated in Slide IV,16, is a giant cell tumor until proved otherwise. A giant cell tumor is typically a lytic, poorly defined metaphyseal-epiphyseal lesion adjacent to the subchondral bone. Note also in Slide IV,16 the pathologic fracture in the posterior cortex of the tibia. In Slide IV,17, the histologic features of a giant cell tumor are seen. These features include random distribution of osteoclast-type giant cells. The large vacuolated nuclei of the stromal cells are similar to the nuclei of the giant cells. In older adults, lesions at the metaphyseal-diaphyseal junction are most likely metastatic carcinoma, as depicted in Slide IV,18. This slide shows an

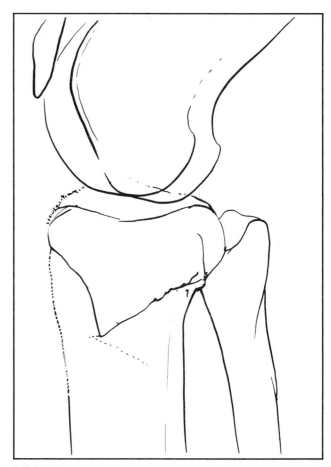

Slide IV,16

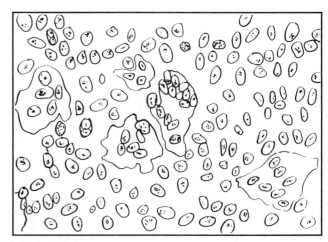

Slide IV,17

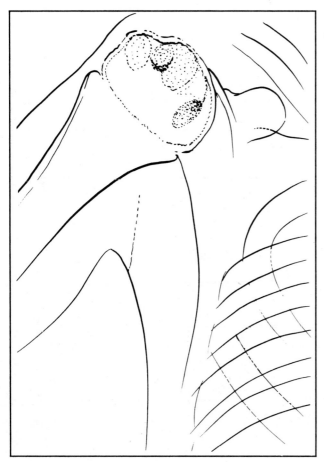

Slide IV,15

anteroposterior radiograph of the proximal femur of a patient known to have a primary lung carcinoma. The diffuse, infiltrating involvement of the diaphyseal-metaphyseal junction with minimal bony reaction is typical of metastatic disease.

The most rapidly growing bone tumors invade the medullary trabecular bone (producing a wide transition zone), permeate the cortex, usually breach the periosteum, and have an associated soft-tissue mass. Slide IV,19 is a diagram illustrating the radiographic features of a highly aggressive bone lesion. A radiograph of the most aggressive pattern is shown in Slide IV,20. These features include diffuse, permeative, poorly defined involvement of the medullary cavity, permeation of the cortex with an associated soft-tissue mass, and focal periosteal reaction. The specific finding of cortical excavation ("saucerization") strongly suggests a Ewing sarcoma rather than other malignant tumors. Slide IV,21

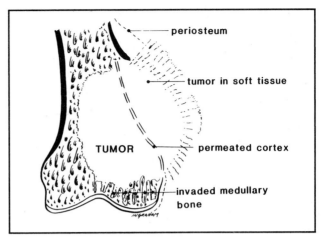

Slide IV,19

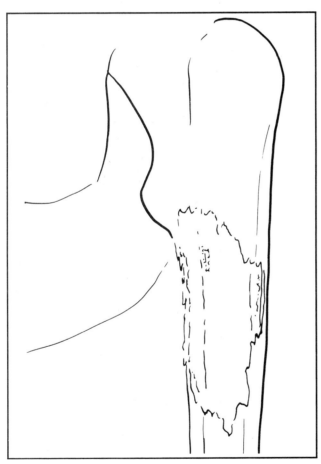

Slide IV,18

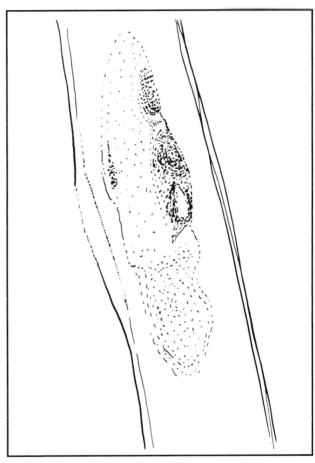

Slide IV,20

shows a histologic section of a Ewing sarcoma. Sheets of a homogeneous population of small round cells with clear cytoplasm and remarkably uniform nuclei with few or no mitoses can be seen. The lack of other cell populations such as lymphocytes and plasma cells rules out the diagnostic choices of infection or eosinophilic granuloma. Slide VI,22 points out the aggressive infiltrative nature of a sarcoma. Note the transgression of the epiphyseal plate through the cortex, penetration of the fibrous periosteum into soft tissue, and irregular loss of medullary cancellous bone with replacement of the marrow by tumor. There are a variety of periosteal reactions associated with aggressive growth patterns. The Codman triangle is the most common and is the result of remaining cortex and benign reactive periosteal bone at the periphery of the lesion. Slide IV,23 is a radiograph illustrating the Codman triangle associated with a highly aggressive sarcoma. Codman's triangles are present proximally, both anteriorly and posteriorly. A different case of highly aggressive sarcoma with soft tissue extension is depicted in Slide IV,24. The Codman triangle is clearly evident proximally. Also note the tumor's periosteal transgression and permeation through the growth plate. The diffuse marrow infiltration signals malignancy. Longitudinal laminated periosteal reaction or "onion skinning" is caused by the tumor's repeated penetration of the benign periosteal reactive bone and can be seen in Slide IV,25. Spicules of tumor bone perpendicular to the cortex, either "hair-on-end" as shown in Slide IV,26 or "sunburst" as in Slide IV,27, are also important clues.

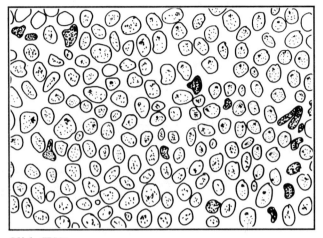

Slide IV,21

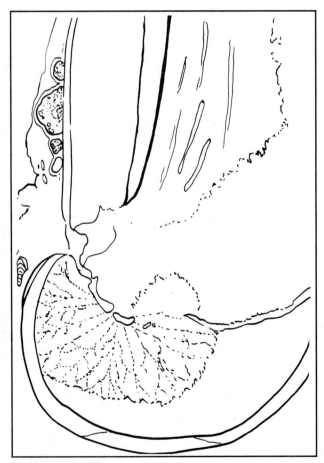

Slide IV,22

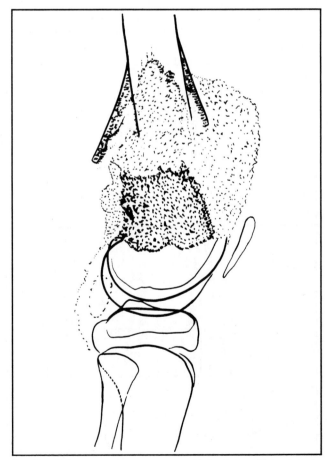

Slide IV,23

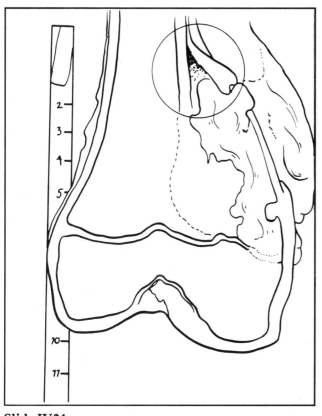

Slide IV,24

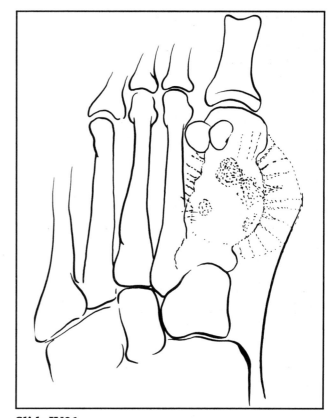

Slide IV,26

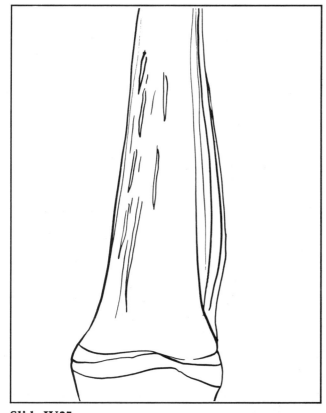

Slide IV,25

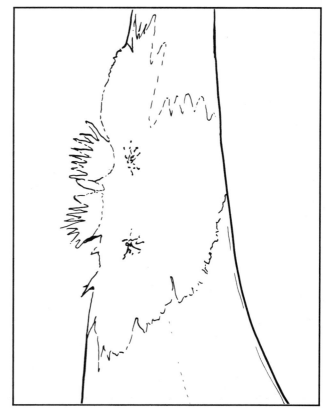

Slide IV,27

Very rapidly growing bone tumors are the most aggressive and are usually malignant. The presence of obvious tumor bone formation is diagnostic of an osteosarcoma and is well illustrated in Slide IV,28, a radiograph of a proximal tibia. Slide IV,29 is a histologic section of an osteosarcoma. A normal segment of lamellar bone (trabecula) is in the center of the slide surrounded by woven bone produced by the sarcoma cells. The neoplastic cells vary in size and shape. Most have large, dark nuclei. A large soft-tissue mass associated with the aggressive radiographic changes strongly suggests a Ewing sarcoma. In Slide IV,30, a Ewing sarcoma is shown involving the left supra-acetabular region extending into the ramus. The laminated "onion-skin" periosteal reaction along the pubis, the poorly defined permeative lucency of the bone, and the loss of subchondral architecture can be observed. A computerized axial tomograph of this same case of Ewing's sarcoma (Slide IV,31) shows the huge size of the soft-tissue mass ("T"), which was not apparent on the plain radiograph. Periacetabular lesions, usually with calcifications, are suggestive of chondrosarcoma. Slide

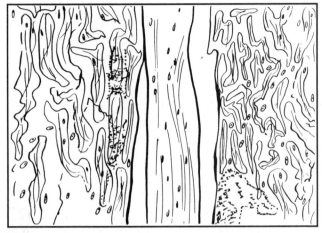

Slide IV,29

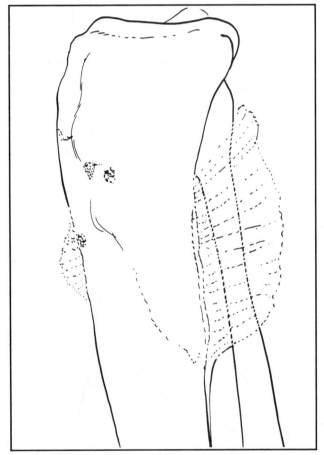

Slide IV,28

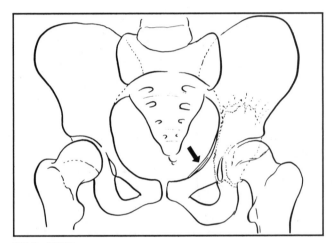

Slide IV,30

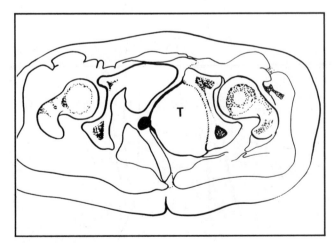

Slide IV,31

IV,32 depicts a high-grade chondrosarcoma involving the periacetabular region. The features of this lesion include lucency, diffusely increased peripheral margins, cortical thinning, and even a soft-tissue mass. Myeloma is the most common primary malignant bone tumor in adults. It usually appears on the radiograph as diffuse osteopenia, or as a radiolucent defect without bone reaction. A solitary radiolucency with a periosteal shell, or rarely an osteoblastic lesion may also be myeloma.

Slide IV,33 shows a lumbar spine radiograph taken because the patient complained of back pain. There is a radiolucent lesion in the sacral wing. The radiographic appearance of a destructive lesion without bony reaction, particularly in a flat bone, is typical of myeloma. The technetium-99 diphosphonate bone scan may not show increased uptake. Patients with myeloma should have a skeletal survey.

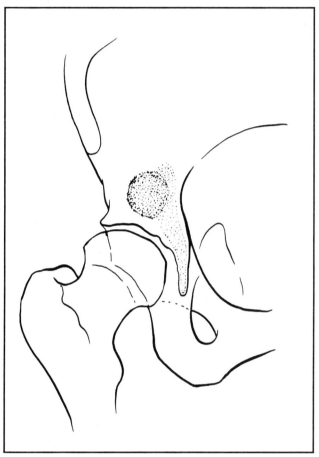

Slide IV,32

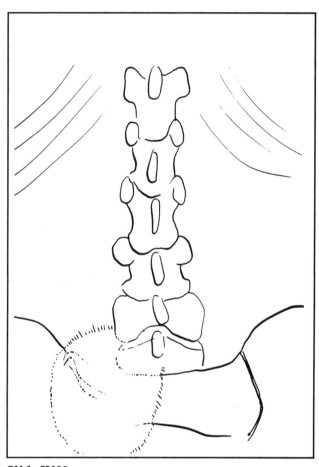

Slide IV,33

Juxtacortical Lesions

Juxtacortical lesions represent a special anatomic site, but the cell of origin may be osteoblastic, chondroblastic or fibroblastic. Juxtacortical lesions do not spontaneously resolve and require surgical resection. Slide IV,34 shows a juxtacortical tumor confined to the cortex and periosteum with local cortical erosion. These lesions should be evaluated thoroughly prior to excision. A lesion often confused with a juxtacortical lesion is an osteochondroma. Osteochondroma is a common, benign, non-neoplastic tumor that usually requires no treatment and should be recognized on the plain radiograph, tomograph, or computed axial tomography. Slide IV,35 shows a radiograph of an osteochondroma with a prominent mineralized cartilage cap and a well-defined stalk in continuity with the underlying marrow cavity of the host bone. Only if this continuity can be demonstrated can the diagnosis be made. Slide IV,36 is a photograph of the gross specimen shown in Slide IV,35. The prominent cartilage cap and the cancellous bone in the stalk in direct continuity with the marrow cavity are clearly seen. Biopsy for diagnosis is inappropriate. Osteochondroma may be solitary or multiple. When multiple, the patient may have a positive family history.

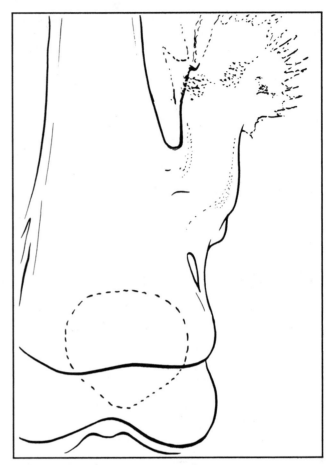

Slide IV,35

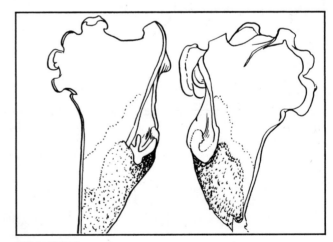

Slide IV,36

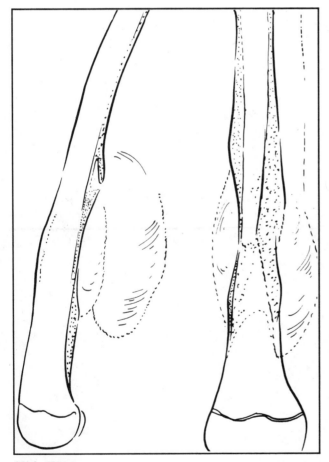

Slide IV,34

Staging

As shown in Slide IV,37, a surgical staging system has been developed for musculoskeletal tumors. This staging system has been adopted by the Musculoskeletal Tumor Society. Lesions are classified as either low grade or high grade based primarily on histologic appearance, but also on clinical presentation. Low-grade tumors have a metastatic potential of less than 25% and are staged as I. High-grade lesions are those with metastatic potential greater than 25% and are staged as II. Any patient who presents initially with metastatic disease is staged a III. The second component of the surgical staging system is whether the lesion is intracompartmental or extracompartmental. Intracompartmental lesions are totally interosseous and are confined to a single anatomic compartment. These are staged as "A." Lesions that have escaped their primary compartment are classified as extracompartmental and are "B" lesions. Thus, the staging system incorporates both the anatomic extent and the histologic and clinical grade. There are six stages in this surgical staging system, as shown on the slide.

STAGE	GRADE	SITE	METASTASIS
IA	Low (G_1)	Intracompartmental (T_1)	None (M_0)
IB	Low (G_1)	Extracompartmental (T_2)	None (M_0)
IIA	High (G_2)	Intracompartmental (T_1)	None (M_0)
IIB	High (G_2)	Extracompartmental (T_2)	None (M_0)
IIIA	Low (G_1) or High (G_2)	Intracompartmental (T_1)	Yes (M_1)
IIIB	Low (G_1) or High (G_2)	Extracompartmental (T_2)	Yes (M_1)

Slide IV,37

In order that physicians may discuss the type of surgical procedures done, surgical margins have been defined, as illustrated in Slide IV,38 top. The types of surgical margins are intralesional, marginal, wide, or radical. The use of this terminology facilitates proper classification and communication of surgical technique.

It is possible to develop basic surgical indications once surgical margins have been defined and the patient has been properly staged, as illustrated in Slide IV,38 bottom. The surgical indications illustrated in this slide are not intended as absolutes, but rather as guidelines upon which specific treatment for individual patients can be based.

SURGICAL MARGINS

TYPE	PLANE OF DISSECTION	RESULT
Intralesional	Piecemeal debulking or curettage	Leaves macroscopic disease
Marginal	Shell out enbloc through pseudo-capsule or normal tissue	May leave either "satellite" or "skips"
Wide	Intracompartment enbloc with cuff	May leave skip
Radical	Extracompartmental—enbloc entire compartmental	No residual

SURGICAL INDICATIONS

MARGIN	LOCAL	AMPUTATION
Intralesional	benign: selfhealing malignant: palliation adjunct to RT or chemotherapy	benign: — malignant: palliation adjunct to RT or chemotherapy
Marginal	benign: persistent malignant: palliation adjunct to RT for stage I	benign: persistent recurrent malignant: adjunct to RT for stage I
Wide	benign: recurrent or aggressive malignant: I-A II-A with adjunctive chemotherapy	benign: aggressive recurrent malignant: I-B II-B with adjunctive chemotherapy
Radical	benign: — malignant: recurrent I-A, II-A	benign: — recurrent I-B, II-B

Slide IV,38

Soft-Tissue Tumors

Intramuscular lipomas are the only benign soft-tissue tumors occurring in adults that can be confidently diagnosed without a biopsy. Slide IV,39 shows a computed axial tomography of a patient with a left axillar mass that has the density of fat. When the entire lesion has the density of fat, the lesion may be confidently diagnosed as a benign lipoma. Subcutaneous lesions may be malignant but usually are not. Therefore, since biopsy contaminates the surrounding tissue, it should not be performed until after the tumor has been thoroughly staged.

All deep soft-tissue tumors should be considered malignant and evaluated as such unless the diagnosis of a benign intramuscular lipoma can be made following computed axial tomography.

Malignant soft-tissue tumors grow by infiltrating the surrounding tissue and therefore are never truly encapsulated. The surrounding normal tissue responds by forming a pseudocapsule, as shown in Slide IV,40. This pseudocapsule is composed of compressed collagen vessels stained pink. The soft-tissue sarcoma is the cellular blue area. Slide IV,41 is a diagram of tumor

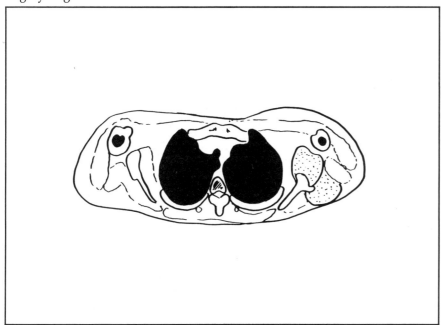

Slide IV,39

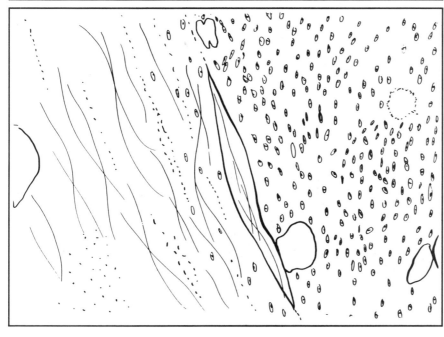

Slide IV,40

invading muscle. The pseudocapsule may be infiltrated by tumor cells and is often completely penetrated. The more aggressive the tumor the more likely the tumor cells will have escaped the pseudocapsule. Slide IV,42 is a gross specimen of a soft-tissue sarcoma with penetration of the pseudocapsule and formation of satellite tumor nodules. Surgical excision through the pseudocapsule ("shell 'em out") leaves tumor cells behind, increasing the risk of local recurrence.

Soft-tissue tumors grow most rapidly in the direction of least resistance and spread longitudinally within the muscle. The muscular fascia acts as a partial barrier to tumor growth. Slide IV,43 shows a gross specimen of tumor permeating muscle without an apparent pseudocapsule. Unless preoperative anatomical localization of the tumor is done, accurate resection margins are impossible. Slide IV,44 is a microscopic section show-

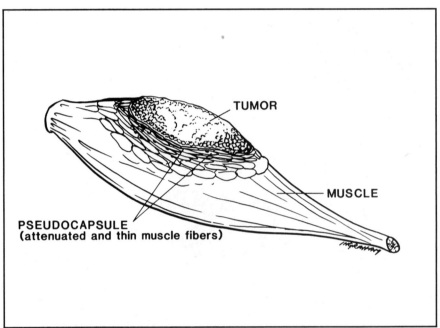

Slide IV,41

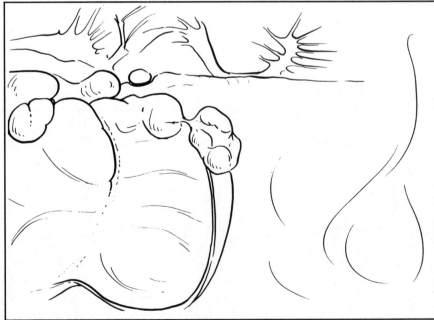

Slide IV,42

ing the pattern of soft-tissue tumor invasion of muscle. The linear strands of pink tissue dissecting between the red skeletal muscle fibers are tumor ("T").

The fascial boundaries between muscle compartments act as even greater barriers to tumor growth but may be penetrated by the most aggressive tumors. Spread of tumor cells out of their muscles of origin takes place across fascial boundaries or into adjacent bone along the normal vascular channels passing from one compartment to the next. Tumor cells will also penetrate reparative scar tissue and will cross surgically disrupted anatomic barriers. The propensity of soft-tissue tumors to grow longitudinally and to be confined by fascial boundaries has lead to the surgical principle of resecting all the involved muscles from their origin to their insertion. Tissues contaminated during the biopsy must also be excised.

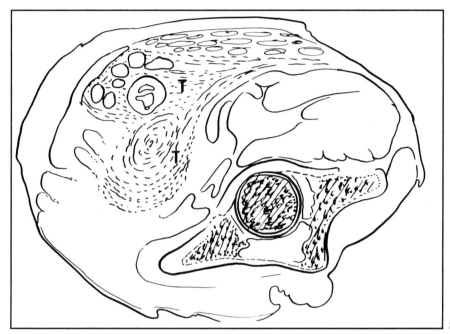

Slide IV,43

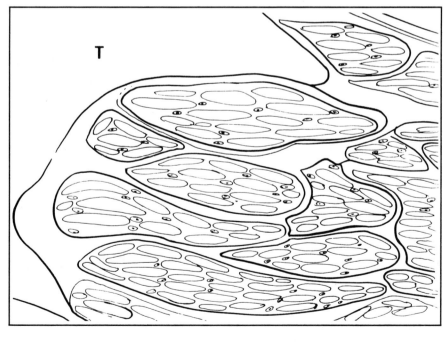

Slide IV,44

Osteomyelitis

Osteomyelitis is an infection of the marrow, trabeculae, and cortex. Although numerous organisms may cause this infection, *Staphylococcus aureus* is the organism most commonly found on culture.

Hematogenous osteomyelitis usually originates in the metaphysis just below the growth plate. The metaphyseal vascular loops are plugged by bacteria and an abscess develops, shown diagrammatically in Slide IV,45. The closed space of the metaphysis and the limited vascular anastomoses predispose to local necrosis of the bone and marrow, permitting the bacteria to resist the host defenses and resulting in a clinical infection. The inflammatory response of the host includes infiltration of acute inflammatory cells and a local vascular proliferation that surrounds but cannot invade the abscess. The host bone attempts to isolate the infection and limit its growth. Slide IV,46 shows a radiograph of the distal tibia with a radiolucent metaphyseal area surrounded by radiodense, poorly defined cortical bone. A focus of lucency crosses the growth plate. The longitudinal tapering of the lucency favors a diagnosis of infection rather than neoplasm. Slide IV,47 is a photomicrograph

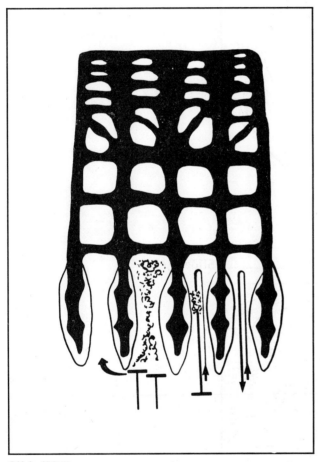

Slide IV,45

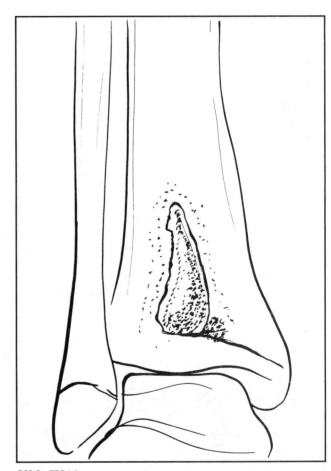

Slide IV,46

of a bone abscess. The marrow is replaced by polymorphonuclear leukocytes (pus) and necrotic lamellar bone (sequestra). Such a focus is characteristic of an early stage of osteomyelitis. Slide IV,48 shows sequential radiographs of a wrist with progressive osteomyelitis. The left panel shows a vague, tapered radiolucency of the radial metaphysis, which represents an early change. The middle panel represents one month's progression:

the pus has extended through the cortex along the vessels and has raised the periosteum to produce a subperiosteal abscess. The underlying necrotic cortex and cancellous bone have formed a sequestrum. The right panel taken 2½ months later, after surgical and antimicrobial therapy, shows a prominent reactive bone response from the periosteum (involucrum) covering the sequestrum.

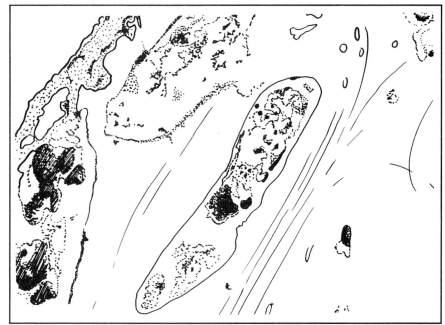

Slide IV,47

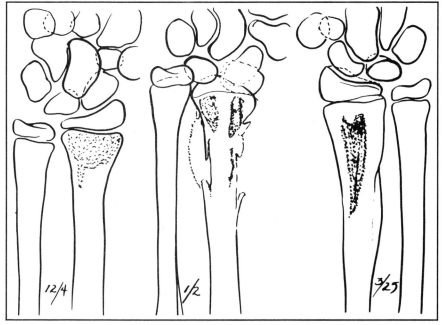

Slide IV,48

If the host is successful in isolating the abscess by means of reactive bone, the patient will have a Brodie abscess. The clinical presentation of a Brodie abscess, often similar to the presentation of a primary tumor, may require a biopsy for diagnosis. The patient should be evaluated as if the lesion were a neoplasm. The elevation of the periosteum is more likely to occur in the child than the teenager or adult because the child's periosteum has fewer perforating vessels and is thicker. Cortical penetration and periosteal elevation are associated with more dramatic clinical findings.

If the abscess goes untreated, the pus will spontaneously decompress by penetrating the periosteum to form a soft-tissue abscess that will eventually drain through the skin. The cutaneous sinus will eventually epithelize. If the sinus continues to drain for many years, a squamous cell carcinoma may develop. Slide IV,49 shows the capsule of a child's normal hip joint to em-

phasize that the growth plate and metaphysis are within the joint capsule. Hematogenous osteomyelitis beginning in the neck of the femur will decompress into the hip joint, creating a pyarthrosis. Slide IV,50 shows a radiograph of the femoral neck in an infant with osteomyelitis. The abscess has spontaneously drained into the hip joint. Note the prominent involucrum involving the proximal portion of the femur and the destruction of the joint. Other joints with intracapsular growth plates may be subjected to the same fate. Slide IV,51 shows an unusual example of long-standing chronic osteomyelitis that has produced a gaping hole called a cloaca. The cloaca opens from the bone into a sinus tract that communicates with the surface of the skin. The bone cortex visible in the cloaca is the original dead cortex that formed an involucrum which has remained unchanged for years. The entire shaft is the involucrum made up of periosteal bone deposited over the years. The numerous holes in the involucrum are new nutrient vascular fo-

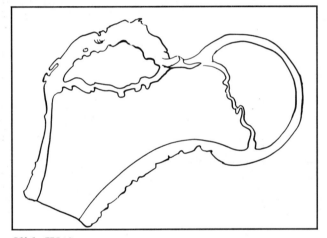

Slide IV,49

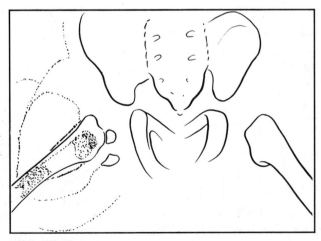

Slide IV,50

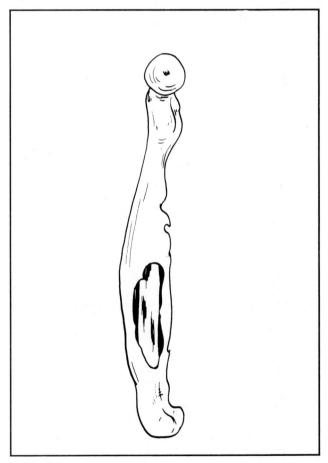

Slide IV,51

ramina to nourish this pseudocortex. Slide IV,52 depicts yet another example of chronic osteomyelitis, with a sequestrum surrounded by an involucrum. Slide IV,53 is a photomicrograph showing chronic osteomyelitis with dead cortical bone being actively resorbed by osteoclasts. The marrow has been replaced by fibrous tissue and chronic inflammatory cells. The photomicrograph in Slide IV,54 shows the new viable woven bone (involucrum) surrounding portions of necrotic fragmented cortex (sequestrum). The cortical fragments are also partially surrounded by inflammatory cells.

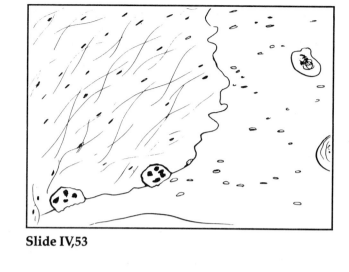

Slide IV,53

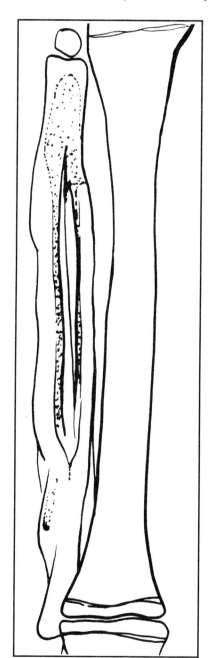

Slide IV,52

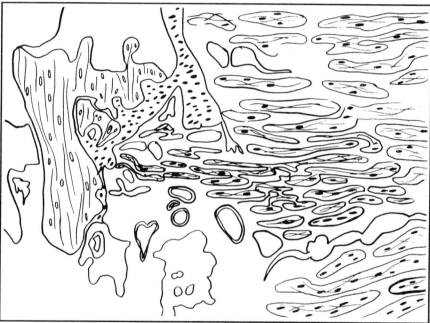

Slide IV,54

Synovial Disease
Rheumatoid Arthritis

Rheumatoid arthritis is a proliferative, autonomous process of synovium that culminates in overgrowth of synovial pannus onto the articular cartilage and into the subchondral bone, with resultant joint destruction, as shown in Slide IV,55. Here we have a photomicrograph of rheumatoid arthritis showing the joint-space obliteration by hyperplastic synovial tissue filled with lymphocytes and plasma cells. There is also a thin pannus covering the articular cartilage as well as pannus erod-

ing the subchondral bone plate and marrow. Rheumatoid arthritis symmetrically involves multiple joints and synovium-lined tendon sheaths. Slide IV,56 is an intraoperative photograph of edematous hyperemic proliferative rheumatoid synovium covering the extensor tendons of the wrist. The radiographic characteristics include juxta-articular osteoporosis, subchondral erosion, and loss of articular cartilage (joint narrowing), all visible in Slide IV,57. The histologic appearance of rheumatoid arthritis and its variants consists of synovial-cell hyperplasia with scattered multinucleated giant cells, surface fibrin deposition, synovial edema, and synovial

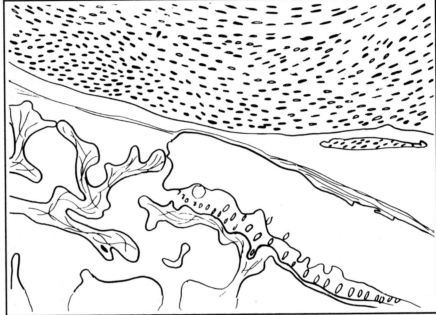

Slide IV,55

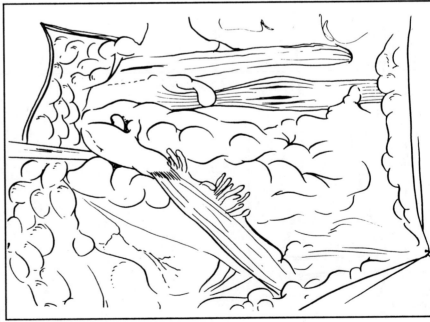

Slide IV,56

papillarity. Furthermore, the synovium is infiltrated by plasmacytic and lymphocytic aggregates sometimes with germinal centers, as shown in Slide IV,58. Slide IV,59 is a photomicrograph of a rheumatoid nodule, rarely found in the synovium, but virtually diagnostic. It is a palisading granuloma with central fibrinoid necrosis.

The pannus in the inflammatory synovium covering the articular cartilage and the "rice" bodies found in the joint are nodules of fibrin. Although a high joint-fluid leukocyte count is characteristic of rheumatoid arthritis, leukocytes are conspicuously absent in the synovium.

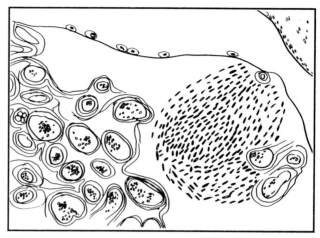

Slide IV,58

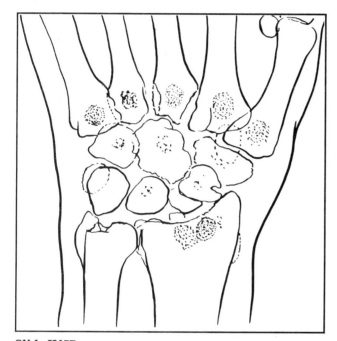

Slide IV,57

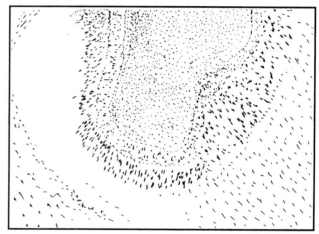

Slide IV,59

Gout

Gout is an inflammatory arthritic disease process secondary to underlying hyperuricemia. In primary gout the hyperuricemia is caused by an inborn error of purine metabolism. The hyperuricemia in secondary gout is commonly seen in patients undergoing chemotherapy for tumors. The acute inflammatory disease affects males more often than females; typically the first metatarsophalangeal joint is involved, as shown in Slide IV,60. There are prominent juxta-articular eccentric bone erosions and a soft-tissue mass, corresponding to the accumulation of sodium urate crystals and adjacent foreign body giant cell reaction. This slide presents a classic example of podagra. The accumulation of sodium urate crystals within the synovium produces a foreign body giant cell reaction and proliferative synovitis with subsequent joint destruction. Slide IV,61 is a whole mount photomicrograph of the case shown in Slide IV,60. The tophus, joint destruction, and even marrow invasion by the reactive tissue are clearly visible.

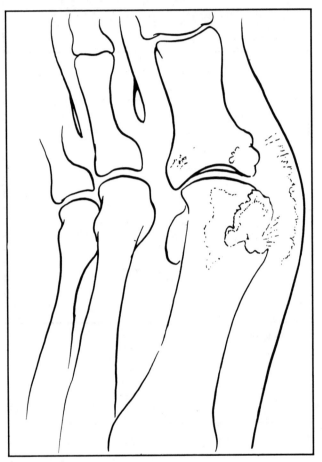

Slide IV,60

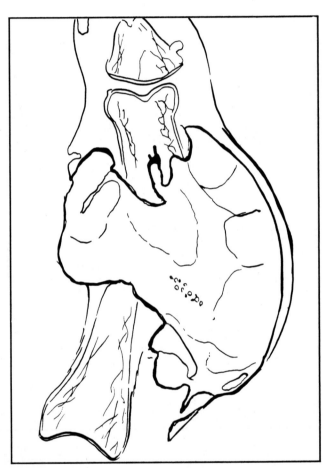

Slide IV,61

A characteristic multinucleate foreign body giant cell reaction to the sodium urate crystals is shown in Slide IV,62. In this preparation, the crystals have been dissolved by histologic solvents, leaving an amorphous proteinaceous fluid. There are also mononuclear inflammatory cells between the giant cells. Finally, Slide IV,63 shows a single urate crystal viewed under polarized light. The crystal has an elongated needle shape and is negatively birefringent in polarized light. Slide IV,64 is presented here to caution the reader regarding granulomatous reactions that may simulate the foreign body giant cell reaction seen in gout. This photomicrograph depicts tuberculosis. Note the clear-cut nodules of large epithelioid cells (histiocytes) and multinucleated giant cells, some of which have a peripheral arrangement of nuclei, typical of the Langhans-type giant cell. Such aggregations of cells form a granuloma. Sodium urate crystals will dissolve if put into a fixative containing water; therefore the chalky white joint fluid should be smeared directly onto the slide and air dried.

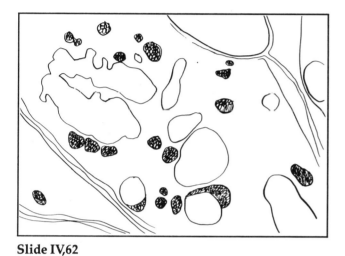

Slide IV,62

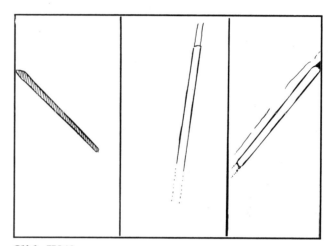

Slide IV,63

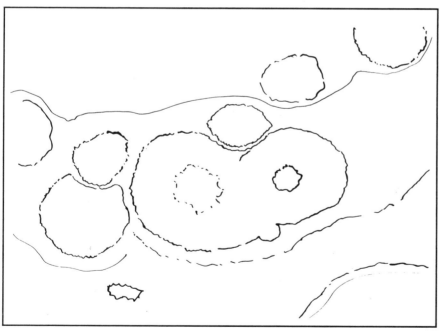

Slide IV,64

Calcium Pyrophosphate Deposition Disease

Calcium pyrophosphate deposition disease (CPDD), or chondrocalcinosis is usually seen in the elderly secondary to the deposit of crystalline materials, most commonly calcium pyrophosphates. As with gout, the pain is secondary to synovial irritation by lysozymes released from the inflammatory cells. The deposition of crystals within the menisci and articular cartilage is the radiographic hallmark of CPDD, as shown in Slide IV,65. In contrast to the sodium urate crystals of gout, calcium in the pyrophosphate crystals of CPDD does not usually invoke a foreign body giant cell reaction. The calcium pyrophosphate crystals are water resistant and can be seen in tissues fixed in formalin or in an alcohol solution. The crystals are short and rhomboid. Slide IV,66 shows the weakly positive birefringent CPP crystal.

Pigmented Villonodular Synovitis

Pigmented villonodular synovitis (PVS) is typically a monoarticular synovial proliferation seen most often in the knee joint of a young adult male. Next most commonly involved is the hip, ankle, or wrist. The patient usually has a painless, bloody effusion. The articular cartilage is usually normal. The proliferating synovium may invade the subchondral bone, producing radiolucent lesions, characteristically on both sides of the joint. Slide IV,67 shows a knee with pigmented villonodular synovitis. Well-defined lytic subchondral lucencies are seen in the tibia and femur. Grossly, the synovium has a reddish-brown, thickened nodular appearance, as shown in Slide IV,68. The synovial nodules distinguish PVS from simple traumatic hemarthrosis.

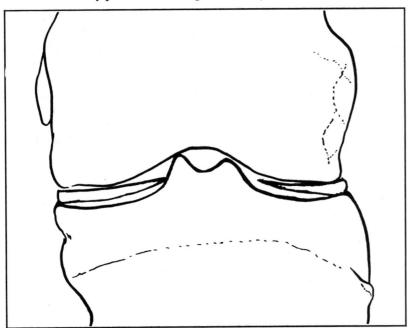

Slide IV,65

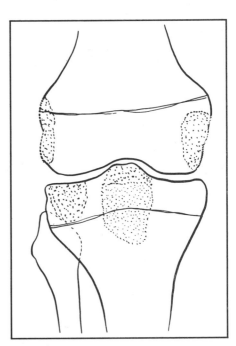

Slide IV,67

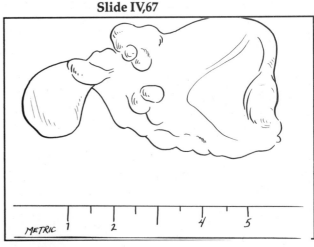

Slide IV,66

Slide IV,68

Synovial Chondromatosis

Synovial chondromatosis is a condition of unknown etiology in which the synovium produces metaplastic cartilage. This cartilage may undergo endochondral ossification to produce a central core of bone, which can be seen on the plain radiograph. When present, the process is called by some synovial osteochondromatosis. Slide IV,69 shows a radiograph of a knee with synovial chondromatosis. Mineralized cartilage nodules are seen posteriorly. However, in some cases there is universal synovial involvement by unmineralized nodules as well as loose bodies ("joint mice"). Since no joint destruction is seen in this radiograph, it is unlikely that loose bodies or a neuropathic joint would be found in this patient. Slide IV,70 presents a typical example of synovial chondromatosis with innumerable cartilage nodules embedded in the synovium. Slide IV,71 is a photomicrograph of a hyaline cartilage nodule of synovial chondromatosis; there is, however, no clear-cut margin between the nodule and adjacent synovial tissue to indicate a metaplastic change. This cartilage nodule may eventually be extruded into the joint as a loose body.

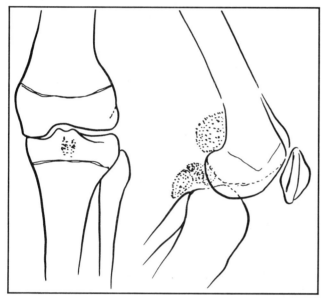

Slide IV,69

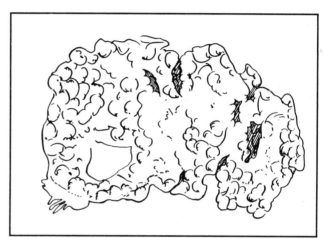

Slide IV,70

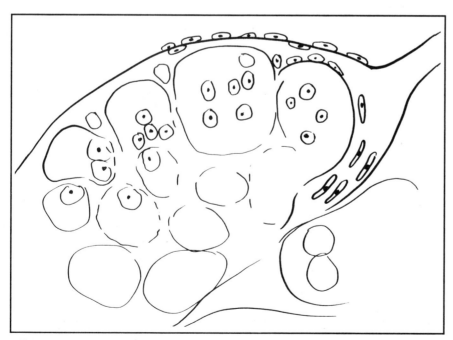

Slide IV,71

Hemophilia

Hemophilia is an X-linked recessive disease seen principally in males. Repeated hemorrhage into major joints stimulates a destructive synovial hyperplasia that leads to synovial hemosiderosis and eventually to a degenerative arthritis. The radiographic characteristics include juxta-articular osteoporosis, a squaring and enlargement of the epiphysis, erosion of bone at the synovial attachments, and loss of articular cartilage, as shown in Slide IV,72. Grossly, the joint shows extensive degenerative changes in the cartilage and deeply black-brown stained hypertrophic synovium, as clearly seen on Slide IV,73.

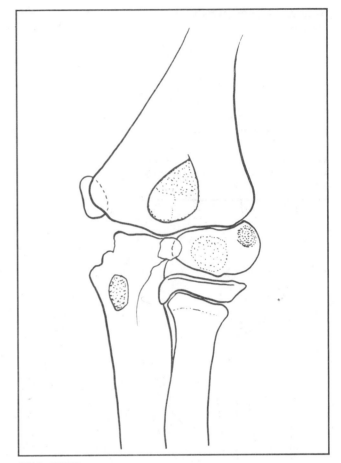

Slide IV,72

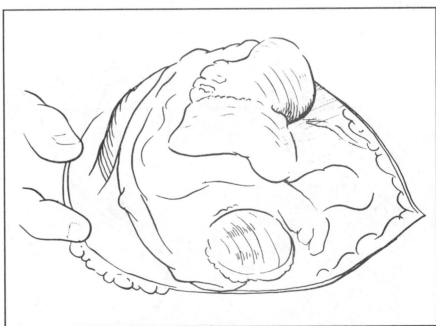

Slide IV,73

Osteonecrosis

Osteonecrosis is a condition in which the marrow and bone are necrotic. Of the many known causes, the most common is a fracture. Other associated factors are corticosteroid therapy, ethanol abuse, alteration of clotting mechanisms, and metabolic diseases (e.g. sickle cell disease, Gaucher's disease). This discussion will emphasize the processes of repairing necrotic bone, which are similar regardless of the cause. The reparative pathways for necrotic trabecular bone and necrotic cortical bone are different, however.

Trabecular Bone and Marrow Osteonecrosis

Necrosis occurs when the blood supply is interrupted. For the sake of simplicity, we can separate the subsequent events into three pathophysiologic steps. In step one, the marrow and trabecular bone tissue die. When the necrosis includes the end of a long bone, the calcified cartilage deep in the tidemark also dies, since its nutrition is supplied by epiphyseal vessels. The dead tissue can be recognized histologically by the loss of marrow cells and the empty osteocyte lacunae. The osteocytes can remain viable within their lucunae for two to three weeks after their systemic nutrition has been disrupted. The radiographic appearance and radiodensities of this area are normal. Slide IV,74 is a photomicrograph showing the hallmark of dead lamellar bone, namely the absence of osteocytes and adjacent necrotic marrow. Note the loose fibrous tissue with a single vascular bud in one portion of the marrow space.

In step two, within a few hours of tissue death polymorphonuclear leukocytes and then mononuclear cells, including lymphocytes and plasma cells, accumulate at the periphery of the necrotic bone. This process continues for a few days. Within the first week, buds of neovascular tissue from the peripheral viable marrow begin to infiltrate the necrotic zone. At this stage, calcification of the necrotic fat may occur. The peripheral viable marrow is replaced by fibrovascular tissue, and the adjacent trabeculae may undergo focal resorption by the numerous, stimulated osteoclasts. Slide IV,75 is a photomicrograph showing the beginning of "creeping substitution" in which dead lamellar bone of the trabecula is coated by living woven and lamellar bone. The fatty marrow is focally dead; there is loose tissue invasion and subsequent osteoblastic activity. Several areas of osteoclastic resorption are visible, although the osteoclasts themselves are absent. Radiographically there may be minimal focal osteoporosis, no change at all, or focal areas of increased density secondary to calcified fatty soaps that result from the necrotic fat in the marrow.

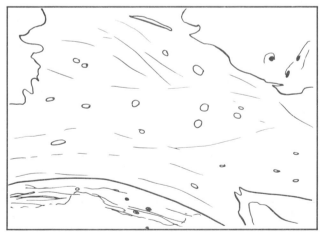

Slide IV,74

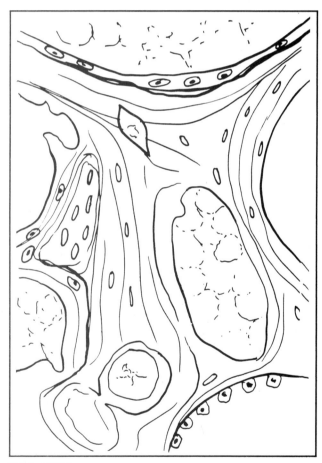

Slide IV,75

In step three of the repair process, some trabeculae remain and some are resorbed. In Slide IV,76 an infarcted trabecula remains and is covered with new lamellar bone produced by the osteoblasts. In other areas, osteoclasts resorb osteonecrotic trabeculae. The resultant radiographic appearance reflects these concomitant biological processes. Radiographs of creeping substitution will therefore show areas of radiolucency (osteoclast activity) and radiodensity (osteoblast activity). In addition to osteoblast activity, other events occur that contribute to the subsequent marked increase in the density of the necrotic bone. Calcification of the necrotic fatty marrow continues. Trabeculae experience fatigue fracture because they cannot respond to stresses

as do viable trabeculae. Collapse and compression of the fractured trabeculae increases their radiodensity. Slide IV,77 shows a corticosteroid-induced bilateral osteonecrosis. All the classic radiographic features are present, including subchondral lucency ("crescent sign"), collapsed and radiodense necrotic zone ("step-off sign"), and a zone of radiolucency adjacent to the necrotic area. Slide IV,78 is a diagrammatic representation of the previous radiograph. The zone corresponding to the empty space represents the crescent sign. Slide IV,79 shows a bisected femoral head with all the areas in the previous diagram outlined. The step-off sign, caused by collapse of the necrotic zone, and the subchondral frac-

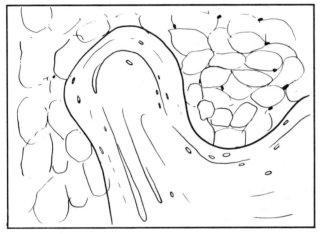

Slide IV,76

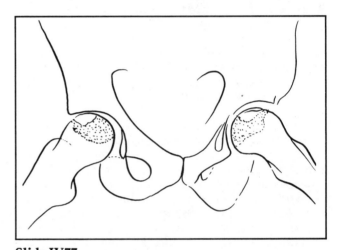

Slide IV,77

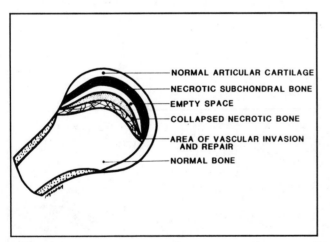

Slide IV,78

NORMAL ARTICULAR CARTILAGE
NECROTIC SUBCHONDRAL BONE
EMPTY SPACE
COLLAPSED NECROTIC BONE
AREA OF VASCULAR INVASION AND REPAIR
NORMAL BONE

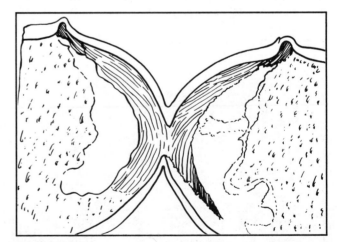

Slide IV,79

ture (crescent sign) are nicely seen here. Slide IV,80 is a photograph of coronal sections through a femoral head with idiopathic osteonecrosis. The black arrows indicate the depth of the necrotic bone, and the subchondral fracture can be easily visualized. The articular cartilage is affected only where the fracture has produced a large wrinkle in the cartilage. At times the articular cartilage and its remaining subchondral cortex may become a free fragment. Slide IV,81 shows an example of such a fragment in the knee. This condition is known as osteochondritis dissecans.

Cortical Osteonecrosis

In step 1 of cortical osteonecrosis, the bone appears to be essentially unchanged. There is no significant inflammatory component associated with necrosis of cortical bone. Necrotic bone initially remains histologically normal. After two or three weeks the dead osteocytes autodigest, leaving empty lacunae. The bone is biomechanically unchanged from its viable status. Its radiographic appearance is normal.

In step 2 the haversian canals are invaded by a new vessel that brings pleuripotential cells to resorb the surrounding necrotic bone. Slide IV,82 shows a cortical cutting cone boring its way into necrotic cortex. The advancing front is comprised of osteoclasts followed by a new population of osteoblasts. The vascular channel with surrounding pleuripotential mesenchymal cells is also prominent. The resorption will extend only to the limit of the osteon and leave the intralamellar bone unresorbed. The cortical bone is weakened during this phase of repair and is radiographically osteopenic. Maximal resorption is thought to require about one year in humans.

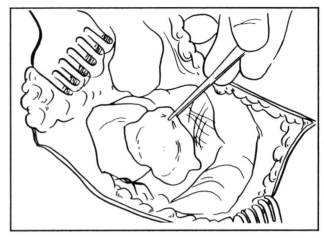

Slide IV,81

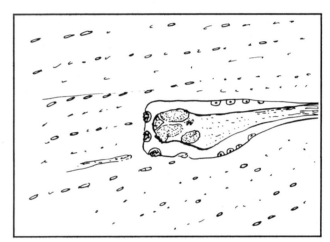

Slide IV,82

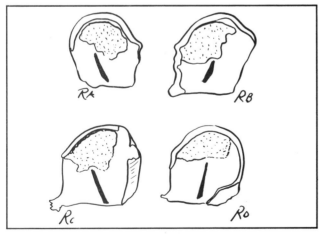

Slide IV,80

In step 3, following resorption, the osteon is replaced by new viable bone. Slide IV,83 shows this later stage. At the end of the cutting cone, new viable woven bone is coating a portion of the dead cortical (lamellar) bone. This process is probably completed about two years after the initial infarction.

The repair and incorporation of bone graft, cancellous and cortical, are essentially identical to the repair of necrotic bone. When cancellous bone is grafted, some cells with osteoblastic potential are also transplanted.

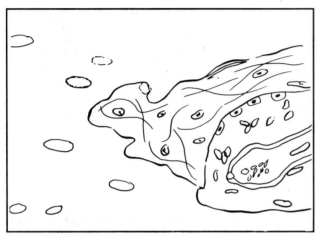

Slide IV,83

Selected Bibliography

Bullough PG , Vigorita JJ: Atlas of Orthopaedic Pathology. Baltimore, Univ Park Press, 1984.

Dahlin DC: Bone Tumors, ed 2. Springfield, IL, CC Thomas, 1981.

Enneking WF, Churchill L: Musculoskeletal Tumor Surgery. New York, Edinburgh, London, and Melbourne, 1983.

Enzinger FM, Weiss SW: Soft Tissue Tumors. St Louis, Toronto, London, CV Mosby, 1983.

Johnston J: Giant cell tumor of bone, the role of the giant cell in orthopedic pathology, in Symposium on Tumors of the Musculoskeletal System. Orthop Clin N Amer 1977; 8:751-770.

Pritchard DJ, Sim FH, Wold LE, et al: Bone tumors, parts I and II. Instructional Course Lectures Vol 33:26-59, 1984.

Springfield DS, Enneking WF, Neff JR, et al: Principles of tumor management. Instructional Course Lectures Vol 33:1-25, 1984.

Symposium in advances in bone tumors, Smith CF, Monsen CG (eds):Clin Orthop Rel Res 1980; 153.

Chapter V

Biomechanics

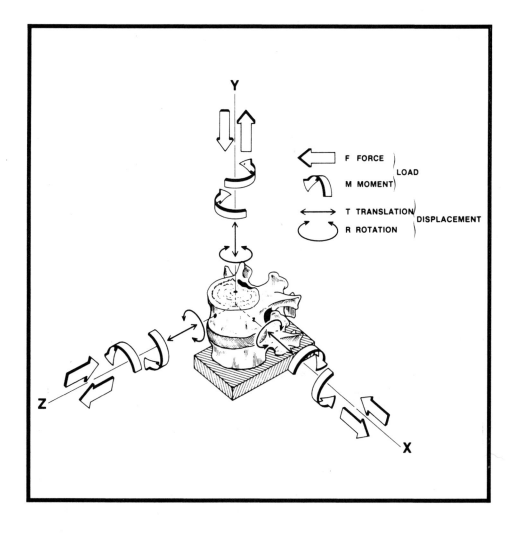

Biomechanics studies the relationship between forces and motions of biologic systems. Rigid body mechanics studies the macroscopic motion of objects, such as extremities and joints. The forces applied are assumed to be large and the objects themselves are assumed not to deform. Deformable body mechanics studies the effects of applied forces on the change in size and shape of objects, such as bone, tendon, or ligament. In this chapter, the relationship between tissue deformation and its internal stresses is examined.

This chapter stresses the principle that the musculoskeletal system, although extremely complex, obeys the basic laws of mechanics. The chapter is divided into the following categories: skeletal forces; biomechanics of materials: musculoskeletal tissues; biomechanics of structures: musculoskeletal organs; biomechanics of pathological processes; and biomechanics of healing and treatment.

Skeletal Forces

Definition of Force

Forces are "pushes" or "pulls." For example, when the heel contacts the floor during the initial portion of stance phase (heel strike), a force is created between the heel and the floor. The heel pushes on the floor and the floor pushes back. Slide V,1 shows the force exerted on the heel. The force has a direction (up) portrayed by the

arrow, as well as a magnitude (790 newtons) represented by the length of the arrow. The force is therefore a vector quantity, since it has both direction and magnitude.

Definition of Moment

The rotating action produced by a force applied to an object is called a "moment." The force applied to the wrench handle in Slide V,2 creates a twisting effect (moment) about the axis of the bolt. The magnitude of the moment is equal to the amount of force multiplied by the perpendicular distance (d) from the axis of the bolt to the line of action of the force. In this case, there is a 200-newton force applied on the handle at a perpendicular distance of 25 centimeters from the bolt. The moment applied to the bolt is therefore 200 n x 25 cm or 5000 n-cm. Note that the unit used to express moment is a combination of the force unit multiplied by the distance unit.

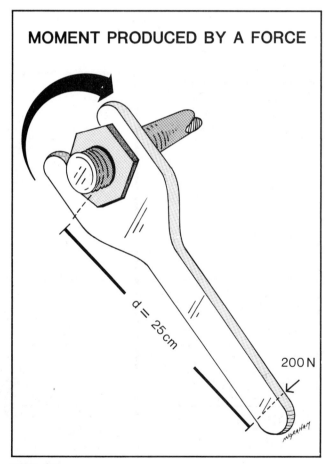

Slide V,2

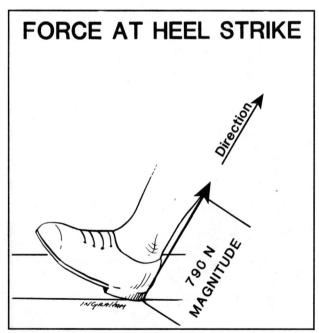

Slide V,1

Definition of Equilibrium

For an object to be in equilibrium, the net effect of all forces and all moments acting on the object must be zero. Slide V,3 illustrates the concept of equilibrium. The amount of force applied at the hinge support of the see-saw must equal the sum of the weight of the two children. The three forces must total to zero: [300 n (down) + 600 n (down)] – 900 n (up) = O.

For an object to be in equilibrium, the sum of all the moments must also equal zero. In this slide, since the see-saw is not rotating, the net moment about the hinge support must equal zero. The 300 n child is sitting 2 meters to the left of the hinge, while the 600 n child is sitting one meter to the right of the hinge. The two moments (300 n x 2 m and 600 n x 1 m) sum to zero because they are in opposite directions. The reaction force of 900 n at the hinge does not cause a moment about the hinge, since the distance between the rotational axis of the hinge and the force (called the moment arm) is zero.

Forces on the Hip Joint

The concept of moment equilibrium can be applied to determine the abductor forces acting about the hip joint. Slide V,4 illustrates the simple case of a person standing on the right leg. The body and the left leg are supported and balanced by the forces acting on the right femoral head. The weight of the body and left leg is ⁵⁄₆ of the total weight (w) of the person. This weight

($\frac{5}{6}$w) will tend to rotate the body about the femoral head and is counteracted by the pull of the abductor muscles on the pelvis. If the body is in equilibrium, the moment created by the abductor muscles must balance the moment created by the gravitational force of $\frac{5}{6}$w. As shown in Slide V,5, the perpendicular distance from the center of the hip joint to the line of action of the $\frac{5}{6}$ body weight is "b" and the perpendicular distance from the center of the hip joint to the abductor muscle force (F_{AB}) is "a." The two moments are ($\frac{5}{6}$w) x (b) and (F_{AB}) x (a). The sum of these two moments must equal zero for the body to be in equilibrium about the hip joint. Given a body weight (w), a measured distance of "a" equal to 5 cm, and a "b" equal to 15 cm, the abductor muscle force (F_{AB}) will be 2½ w. Notice that the reaction force at the joint (Fj) does not create a moment about the joint center (center of rotation) similar to the reaction force at the hinge in the see-saw.

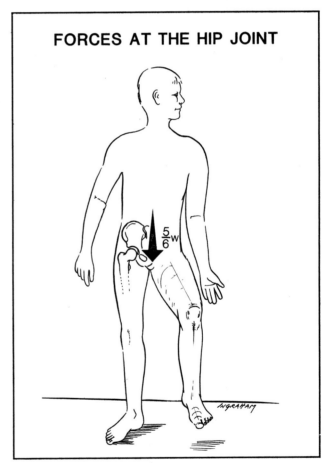

FORCES AT THE HIP JOINT

Slide V,4

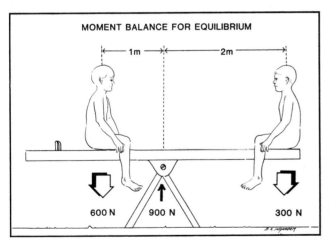

MOMENT BALANCE FOR EQUILIBRIUM

600 N   900 N   300 N

Slide V,3

The hip-joint reaction force can be measured by applying the equilibrium concept that the sum of all forces acting on the hip joint must equal zero. This measurement is made by using a "force triangle" (Slide V,5, right side). When there are only three forces acting on a body in equilibrium, these forces must form a triangle. Since two sides of the triangle are known, the force of gravity on the body ($\frac{5}{6}$w) and the abductor muscle force ($2\frac{1}{2}$w), the triangle can be drawn to scale. The joint reaction force (Fj) equals $3\frac{1}{4}$w, determined by measuring the length of the line. Notice that both the muscle force and the joint reaction force are considerably greater than the weight of the body and leg they are supporting.

Load on Spine

Slide V,6, illustrates the increase in spinal compressive forces caused by holding a weight (W) in the outstretched hand. In this case, the compressive force (F) in the spine can be determined by considering moment equilibrium about a point that lies on the extensor force (F_E). The moment that the weight force (W) creates about the chosen point is (W) x (a+b). The moment that the spinal compressive force increment (F_C) creates about the same point is (F_C) x (a). Since these two moments must balance: $F_C = W(a+b)/(a)$. For a 100 n weight and for an "a" of 5 cm and a "b" of 50 cm, F_C equals 1100 n, or about 11 times the weight lifted.

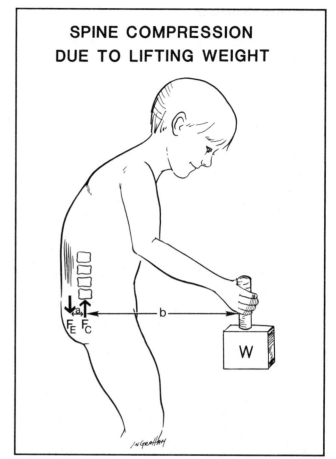

SPINE COMPRESSION DUE TO LIFTING WEIGHT

Slide V,6

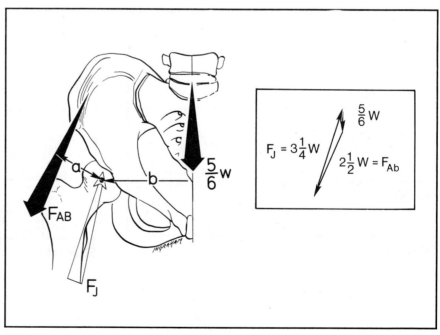

Slide V,5

Forces on the Shoulder

Slide V,7 shows how the muscle and joint reaction force acting about the shoulder can be calculated when a weight is held at arm's length. The muscle force will originate from the deltoid muscle (F_D); the joint reaction force (F_J) is the compressive force between the glenoid fossae and the humeral head. When the arm is in equilibrium, three major forces are acting: the gravity force of the weight W = 100 n; the tension force of the deltoid (F_D); and the compressive force on the humeral head (Fj). Note that the weight of the arm, about 30 n, is ignored; only the increase in forces about the shoulder caused by the weight is calculated.

The deltoid muscle force is determined by summing all the moments about the center of the joint (the center of the humeral head). At equilibrium, the moments must equal zero: [w x 60 cm + (−Fd) x 5cm = 0]. Therefore, the deltoid muscle force (F_D) equals 1½ W, about 1.5 times the average body weight.

The joint reaction force can be found by using the concept of a "force triangle" shown in the lower right hand side of the slide. By drawing the sides of the triangle proportional to the length of the direction of the forces, the joint reaction force (F_J) is found to be 1150 n.

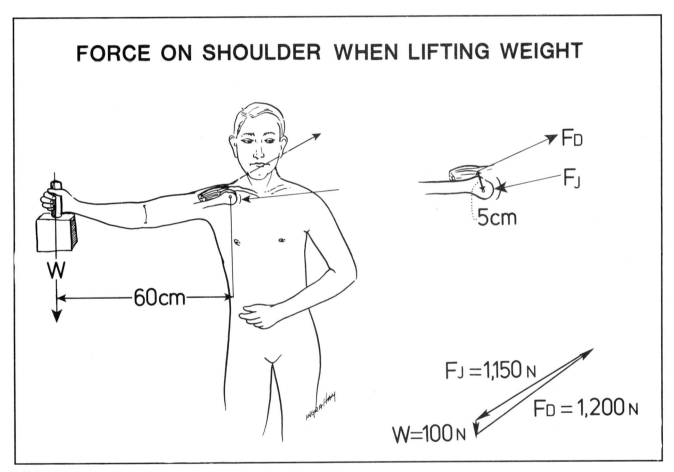

FORCE ON SHOULDER WHEN LIFTING WEIGHT

W

60cm

5cm

F_D

F_J

FJ =1,150 N

FD =1,200 N

W=100 N

Slide V,7

Force on Knee Joint

If a person is slowly climbing steps and stops for an instant, the leg is considered to be in static equilibrium, as shown in Slide V,8. The floor is pushing up on the foot with a force equal to body weight; otherwise the body would be falling. This ground reaction force passes posterior to the knee joint, creating a flexion moment about that joint. For the leg to be in equilibrium, three major forces must be acting: the ground reaction force (W), the tension on the patellar tendon (Fp) and the compressive force on the joint (Fj). To have moment equilibrium about the center of the knee joint, the flexion moment caused by the ground reaction force (W x 7½ cm) must equal the extension moment caused by the patellar tendon force (Fp x 2½ cm). The value for the patellar tendon force (Fp) is 3 W.

By using the force triangle, the joint reaction force is determined to be 3½ W. Thus, large forces can be created at the knee during stair-climbing and other ordinary activities.

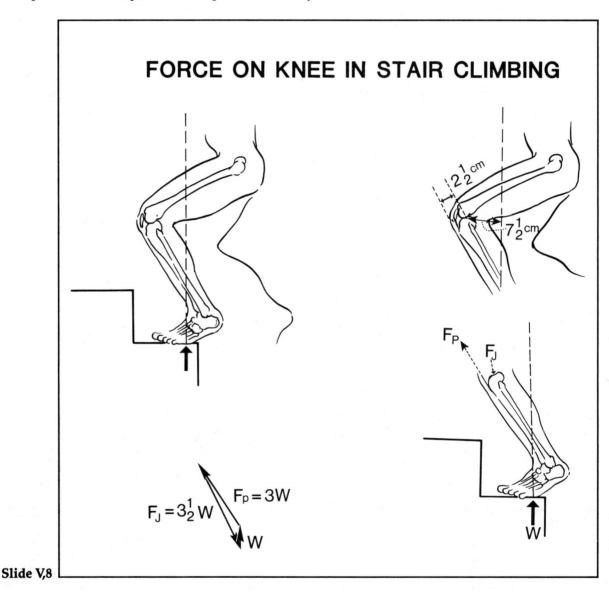

Slide V,8

Force on the Ankle

When a person does a bilateral toe raise, large forces are generated on the ankle. One-half of the body weight (W/2) is supported by each foot. As illustrated in Slide V,9, the ankle dorsiflexion moment created by the ground reaction (W/2 + 16 cm) is balanced by the plantar flexion moment created by the tension of the Achilles tendon (F_A + 4 cm). The moment arms for both of these forces were obtained from radiographic measurement. If these two moments are equal, then the tension (F_A) in the tendon must be 2 W.

Since the tendon force and the ground reaction are both vertical, the joint reaction force can be found by summing the forces in the vertical direction and setting the sum equal to zero (for equilibrium). Thus, the joint reaction must equal the ground reaction (W) plus the tendon force (F_A). F_J then equals 2½ W.

Definition of Translation and Rotation

The motion of any object, in particular any bone, can be described in terms of a combination of linear motion and angular motion. Linear motions, as measured by the distance a point travels, are called "translations." Angular motions, as measured by the change in angular orientation of a line, are called rotations. Six possible motions can be imposed upon bone. As illus-

trated in Slide V,10, the vertebral body can translate in the anteroposterior direction, the lateral direction, or the axial direction. At the same time, the vertebral body can rotate about the flexion-extension axis, the lateral bending axis, or the longitudinal axis. These six possible motions are described as "six degrees of freedom."

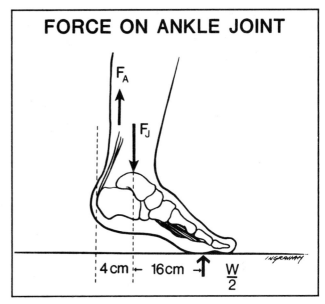

Slide V,9

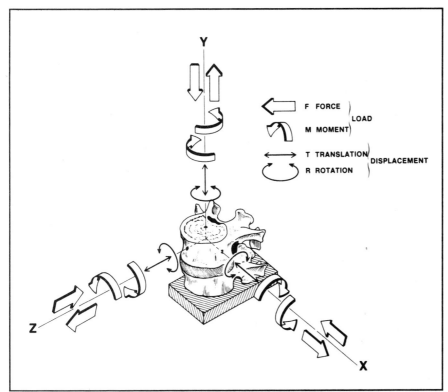

Slide V,10

Relative Motion at Contacting Surfaces

When two objects are in contact and the contact surfaces are neither separating to form a gap nor penetrating to crush one or both objects, the surfaces are in sliding contact or in rolling contact. In rolling contact, the contacting points on the two surfaces have zero relative velocity, while in sliding contact, *some* relative velocity can be measured. These conditions are illustrated by the automobile tire in Slide V,11. When moving across the road, if the tire leaves a clear track or print at the point of contact (the bottom of the tire and the road surface), the relative velocity between the tire and the road is zero; otherwise the print would smear. When a tire rolls, the contact points have zero relative velocity, the axle moves relative to the road at the velocity of the car, and the top of the tire moves relative to the road at twice the velocity of the car.

A similar situation exists when a person walks. The sole of the shoe is in rolling contact with the ground (zero relative velocity between shoe and ground at the contact point). Sliding occurs when the velocity of the contact point is not zero, and the two contact surfaces are undergoing relative motion in a parallel direction. Under these conditions, the tire would leave a skid mark and the shoe would likewise smear its print. Walking or driving on ice frequently results in skidding or sliding. Joint motion consists of both rolling and sliding motion. In most large joints, rolling motion predominates, while in some smaller joints, or where instability exists, sliding motion can become an important factor.

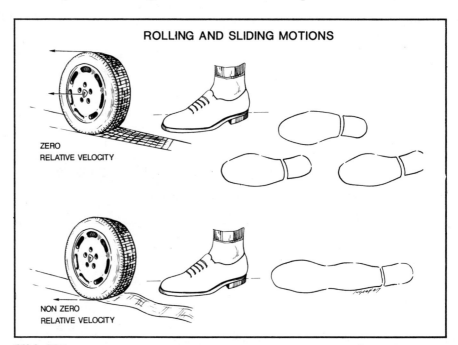

Slide V,11

Biomechanics of Materials: Musculoskeletal Tissues

Definition Of Stress

Stress is defined as force per unit area ($\sigma = F/A$) When forces are applied to a bone, internal forces are produced within the bone. A discussion of stresses within an object can be simplified by considering only the stresses on an imaginary cube within the object. Slide V,12 illustrates a femur being subjected to several forces and depicts the stresses that act on an imaginary cube within the diaphysis. The top face of this cube may be subjected to two types of stresses. The first type of stress, called "normal" stress (σ), is generated by a force (F) acting perpendicular to the surface (A). Normal stress is equal to F/A. The second type of stress is a "shear" stress (t). This shear stress is generated by a force (S) oriented parallel to the surface and is equal to S/A. Normal stress can be either compressive or tensile in nature. The accepted units for both normal stress and shear stress are newtons/m² or Pascal (Pa). (1 newton = 0.225 lb force; 1 Pa = 6895 psi). Stresses are often expressed in terms of megapascals or gigapascals: MPa = Pa x 10³; GPa, = Pa x 10⁶.

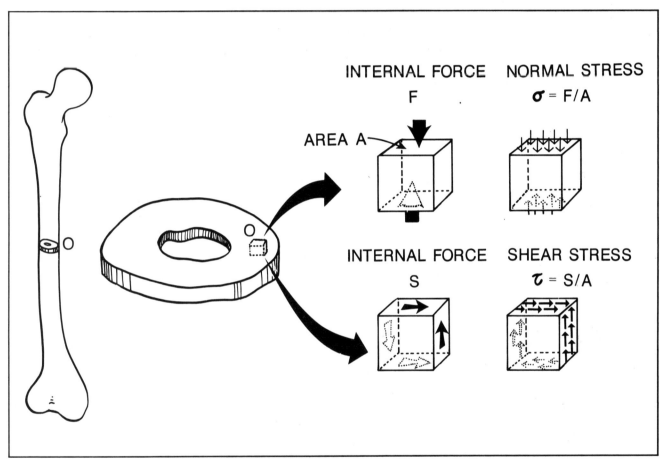

Slide V,12

Definition of Strain

A "normal" strain is produced by a "normal" stress and is defined as the ratio of the change in length ($\triangle$l) of the side of the cube (b) to the original length (l_o) of the side ($\Sigma_s = \triangle l/l_o$). The definition of strain is illustrated in Slide V,13.

A shear stress generated on the top face of the cube causes the front face to deform from a square into a parallelogram. The shear strain is defined as the angular deviation of one side of the cube from its original right angle (expressed in radians). The magnitudes of the normal and shear strains experienced by the cube are influenced by the magnitudes of the stresses as well as by the inherent material properties of the bone tissue. In well mineralized bone, for instance, the tissue is very rigid and small strains result. Conversely, soft tissues are more compliant and thus exhibit much larger strains when subjected to the same degree of stress as bone.

Material Versus Structural Behavior

Because of the complex shapes and loading patterns that occur throughout the skeleton, stresses and strains vary for each bone. In order to concentrate on the mechanical behavior of bone as a tissue (as opposed to the behavior of a whole bone as an organ), it is useful to eliminate the influence of the complex geometry of whole bones. To illustrate this point, imagine a small cylinder of length (l) and cross-sectional area (A) that has been machined from the diaphysis of the femur. The cylinder is subjected to tension forces (F) at each end. Because of the regular geometry of the cylinder, this loading condition results in a uniform pattern of stresses and strains throughout the cylinder at any transverse cross-section. As load is applied, the cylinder begins to stretch. The relationship between the applied force (F) and the increase in length of the bar ($\triangle$l) can be demonstrated by using the example of a spring. Intuitively, the elongation ($\triangle$l) is directly proportional to the applied force (F) and the original length (l_o) and inversely proportional to the cross-sectional area (A) and the stiffness of the material (E).

This can be expressed as follows: $\triangle l = l_o \times F/A \times E$. The stiffness of the material (E) is called Young's modulus. A very stiff material such as steel has a high modulus, and a very deformable material such as rubber has a low modulus. The combination of the geometric parameter (area, A) and the material parameter (modulus, E) is referred to as the axial rigidity (AE) of the cylinder. This factor (AE) expresses the combined effect of both the geometry and material type on the force-length behavior of the cylinder and is one example of structural behavior. The structural behavior of the cylinder can be illustrated as a force-deformation plot (Slide V,14). The linear region (also known as the elastic region) is from O-Y. At Y, "yielding" occurs, with internal rearrangement of the structure, often involving damage to the material. In the region Y-U, non-elastic deformation occurs until finally, at U, fracture results.

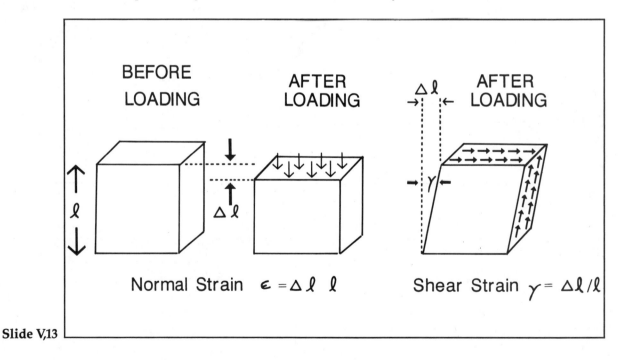

Slide V,13

Because the force-deformation plot changes for cylinders of different cross-sectional areas, it is difficult to use a force-deformation curve (Slide V,14, middle) to represent the behavior of bone. To eliminate this effect of geometry on force-deformation behavior, the force is divided by the cross-sectional area (F/A) and the change in length by the original length ($\triangle l/l_o$). The force-deformation plot then becomes stress-strain plot (Slide V,14, right). This relationship is not affected by the geometry of the cylinder; it simply describes the behavior of the material composing the cylinder. The stress-strain curve represents material behavior, whereas the force-deformation curve represents structural behavior. The key difference is that structural behavior includes the combined effects of geometry and material, while material behavior eliminates the effect of geometry.

In the stress-strain curve, the slope of the linear elastic region has been defined as Young's modulus, E. Since the modulus is defined as the slope of the stress-strain curve in the elastic region and since the units of strain are non-dimensional, the units of modulus are the same as those of stress, MPa or GPa. As shown in the right side of Slide V,14, at Y' the material yields at a stress level known as the yield strength (in units of MPa). At U' the material fractures at a stress level known as the fracture strength or ultimate tensile strength (units of MPa). Note that the stress-strain representation can compare different materials in terms of the elastic modulus, the yield strength, and ultimate strength.

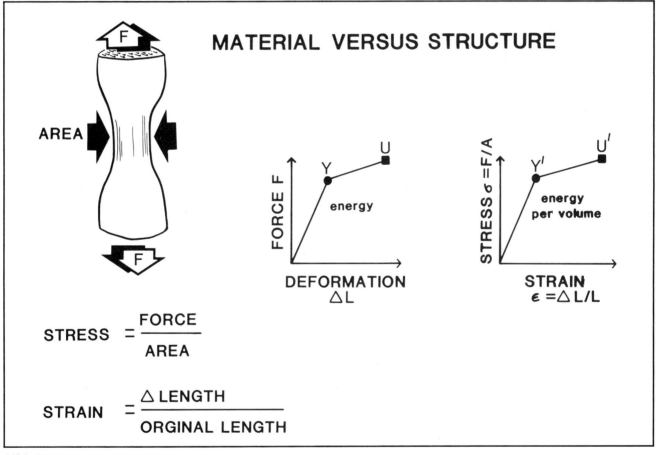

Slide V,14

Cortical Bone: Directional Properties

The stress-strain behavior of cortical bone is largely determined by the orientation of the bone specimen and the direction and type of loading. As shown in Slide V,15, the ultimate strength of cortical bone in the adult femur depends on the orientation of the specimen and on the method of loading (tension, compression or shear). In the longitudinally oriented specimen, the ultimate strength is greatest in compression and lowest in shear. In the transversely oriented specimen, the ultimate strength in tension, compression, and shear is less than their respective strengths in the longitudinally oriented speciman. Cortical bone is more resistant to tension parallel to the predominant orientation of the osteons than it is to tension perpendicular to the osteons. Bone is also stronger in compression than in tension in both a longitudinal and a transverse orientation. Bone is weakest in shear, with the ultimate strength in shear about one-half of the ultimate strength in tension and about one-third the ultimate strength in compression for the longitudinally oriented specimen. The effect of orientation on the strength properties of bone is significant in determining the fracture characteristics of whole bones.

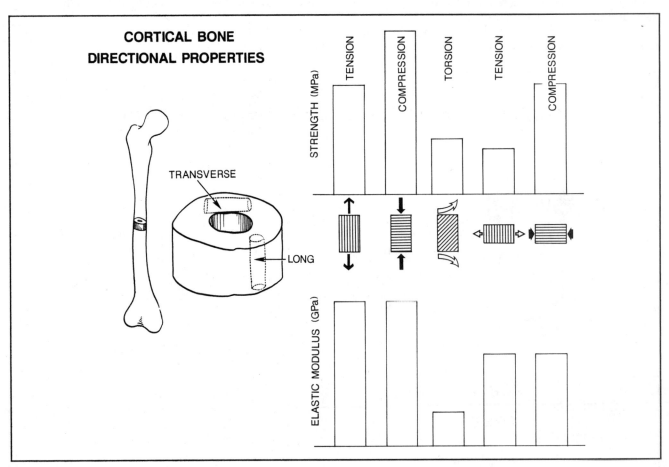

Slide V,15

Cortical Bone: Fatigue Failure

Cortical bone can fracture when exposed to a single, traumatic force. However, cortical bone is also exposed *in vivo* to repetitive stress levels less than those required to fracture the bone during a single, traumatic episode. Repeated loading of bone in daily activities or strenuous exercise may lead to microscopic damage. If damage accumulates faster than it can be repaired by biological processes, a fatigue crack may occur; eventually, it can go on to complete fracture of the bone.

The fatigue behavior of cortical bone can be investigated by subjecting a cylindrical specimen of bone to cyclic tensile strains. Under these test conditions, the fatigue failure process is most sensitive to the strain range (the difference between the maximum and the minimum tensile strain applied to the specimen). At a very large strain range (approximately two times the static yield strain), the bone specimen fails after only a few cycles of applied deformation. At a lower strain range, the specimen may undergo many thousands of deformation cycles before failure.

Slide V,16 shows the strain range plotted against the number of cycles to failure for specimens of cortical bone subjected to cyclic tensile deformation *in vitro* (circles). The slide shows the typical increases in number of cycles to failure for bone specimens subjected to decreasing strain ranges. Also shown are estimates of the strain ranges that occur *in vivo* with normal walking, mild exercise, and very vigorous exercise (broken horizontal lines). The number of deformation cycles that would occur in jogging 10, 100 and 1000 miles is shown by the vertical arrows to the right. This information suggests that the strain ranges necessary to cause fatigue failure of cortical bone *in vitro* are about twice those that occur during very rigorous exercise. It is not surprising that fatigue fractures can occur when neuromuscular control mechanisms are impaired or when the charateristics of the foot-ground contact change with worn running shoes or particularly hard surfaces.

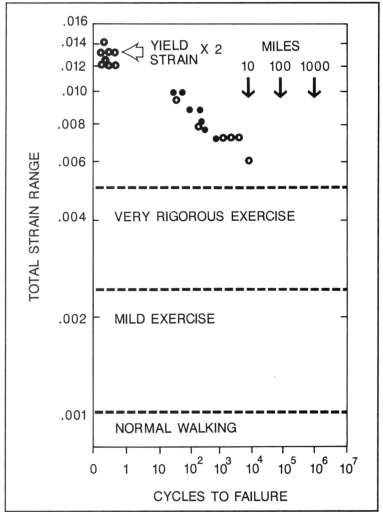

Slide V,16

Trabecular Bone: Effect of Apparent Density

The major physical difference between trabecular bone and cortical bone is the high degree of porosity exhibited by trabecular bone. This degree of porosity can be determined by measuring the apparent density, i.e., the mass of bone tissue divided by the bulk volume—including mineralized bone and bone marrow spaces. In the human skeleton, the apparent density of trabecular bone ranges from 0.1 g/cm to 1 g/cm. The apparent density of cortical bone is about 1.8 g/cm.

Slide V,17 indicates that the compressive strength of all bone tissue in the skeleton is approximately proportional to the square of the apparent density ($\sigma \rho^2$), and the elastic modulus of all bone tissue is approximately proportional to the cube of the apparent density ($\sigma \rho^3$). The effect of age on the strength of bone appears most related to its density; as shown in Slide V,18, the tensile properties of human femoral cortical bone as a material are altered little with increasing age. These relationships between mechanical properties and the apparent density of bone tissue are important, both physiologically and biomechanically. First, they indicate

that bone tissue can change in both modulus and strength as a result of small changes in apparent bone density. The squared and cubic relationships shown in the slide indicate that such reductions in bone density result in very large reductions in bone stiffness and strength.

Ligaments and Tendons: Material Properties

The mechanical properties of soft tissues, such as ligaments and tendons, are significantly different from the mechanical properties of bone. The load-deformation curve for a ligament or tendon is seen in Slide V,19. At the onset of loading, the curve is nonlinear and concave upward in the toe region. The collagen fibers in a ligament or tendon straighten, losing their crimp, and require progressively more stress to elongate. In the linear region, the slope of this portion of the load-deformation curve becomes the steepest and ends by the failure of some collagen fibers. With further elongation, complete failure occurs at strain levels much higher than those of bone: e.g., 8%-10% for flexor digitorum profundus tendon; 12%-15% for medial collateral ligaments; and even higher for cruciate ligaments.

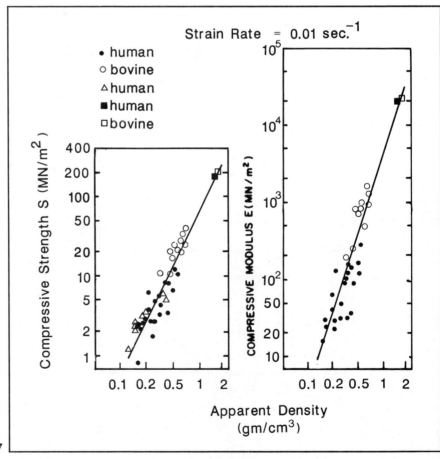

Slide V,17

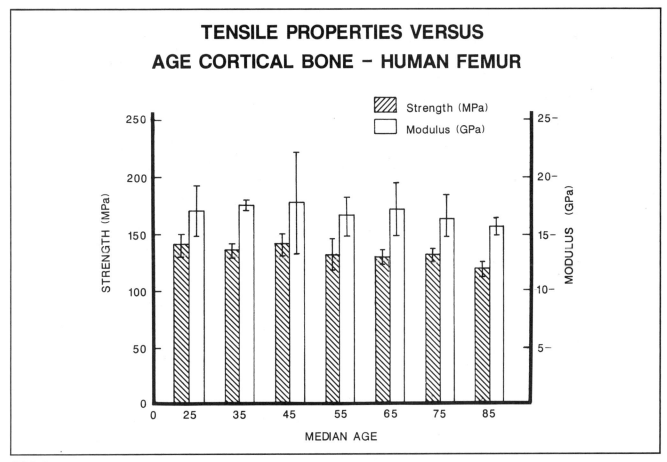

Slide V,18

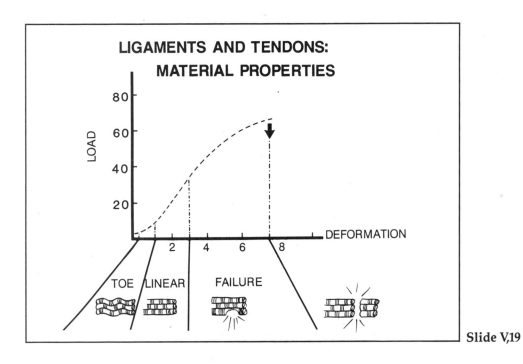

Slide V,19

Material Properties of Various Soft Tissues

The properties of several types of soft tissues are shown in Slide V,20. Their load-deformation curves vary widely, with digital tendons being the stiffest material and skin being the least stiff. Little or no stress is required to deform some animals' dorsal skin to 70% strain, or 1.7 times its original length. The load-deformation curves for ligament and articular cartilage lie somewhere in between these two extremes. The organization of the collagen fibers is largely responsible for the differences in properties of various soft tissues. When magnified under polarized light, the collagen fibers of a tendon specimen are in parallel alignment but exhibit a wavy pattern. During tensile deformation (elongation), the number of fibers being straightened is gradually increased, thus resulting in greater stiffness. As a result, the stress-strain curve is nonlinear and rapidly becomes concave upwards. These densely packed parallel fibers are well suited for the functional demands put on tendon, i.e., to offer early and increasing resistance to tensile loads with a relatively limited amount of deformation, yet sufficient to permit needed joint mobility.

In contrast to tendon fibers, skin fibers appear randomly oriented when viewed under polarized light.

When a skin specimen is subjected to very small tensile forces, a large amount of deformation occurs because of the fiber realignment. Once the fibers are realigned, stiffness of skin increases rapidly, and its behavior becomes similar to that of fibered tissues with parallel alignment, such as tendons.

Bone-Ligament Complex: Material Properties

Slide V,21 depicts the mechanical properties of the anterior cruciate ligament exhibited during a tensile test to failure of a femur-ligament-tibia functional unit. The rate of loading used is moderately high. The failure sequence of this ligament-bone structure, as depicted in the upper portion of this slide, can be correlated with the force-deformation curve. The tensile test starts with relatively large deformation and correspondingly small forces (region 1). At larger ligament forces, (region 1-2), microfailure of fibers occurs, and eventually a force and elongation are reached at which a drop in force will take place, reflecting possible failure of a few collagen fiber bundles. At this point, if the structure is unloaded, the ligament will appear grossly intact but lax, as significant damage has been done to its fibers. With further loading (region 2-3), more fibers are elongated and the

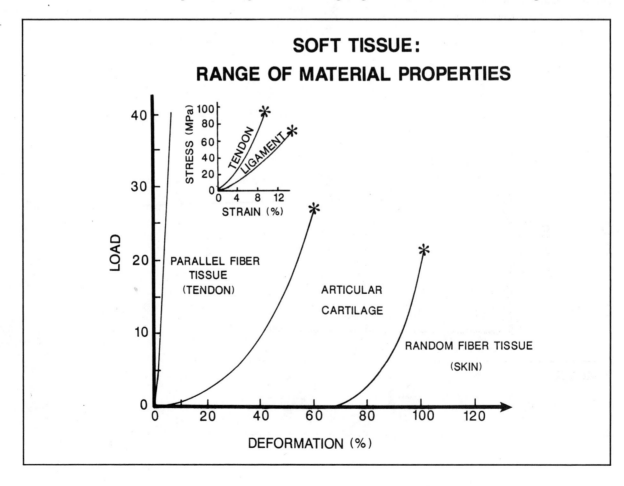

Slide V,20

force continues to rise until a maximum is reached. Finally, complete disruption occurs and the structure loses its load-bearing ability (region 3-4). Although the structure is supporting no load at this stage, the anterior cruciate ligament can, in many instances, appear to be continuous because its synovial lining remains intact.

Ligament Trauma: Effects of Strain Rates

As shown in Slide V,22 the rate of loading plays a significant role in the modes of failure of a bone-ligament-bone functional unit, in part due to the different mechanical properties of bone and ligament at different loading rates. During slower rates of loading, a large percentage of failures will be avulsion type, either at the ligament insertion into bone or to bone. During rapid rates of loading, a high percentage of ligaments will fail within their substance, and the level of force required for failure of the structure is generally higher than the force required for failure at slower rates.

For most soft tissues (including ligaments), strain-rate sensitivity is slight, i.e., the mechanical properties do not change over several decades of changes in the rate of loading. In contrast, strain-rate sensitivity of bone is clearly demonstrable, i.e, the strength of bone increases severalfold over a few decades' increase in

strain rates. Thus, at low loading rates, bone fails because it is weaker in tension than tendon; and at higher loading rates, while the strength of tendon does not change, bone is significantly stronger than tendon.

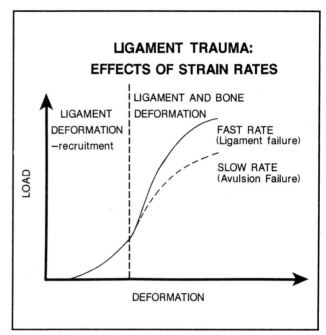

Slide V,22

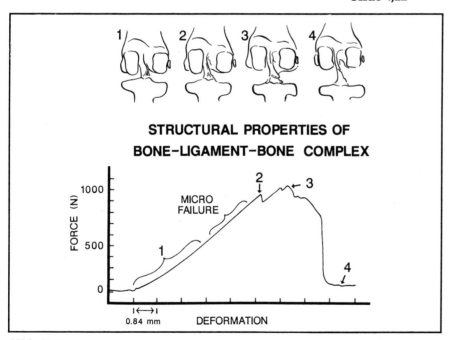

Slide V,21

Meniscus: Directional Properties

The tensile properties of the meniscus are controlled by the architectural arrangement of the collagen network. The surface layers of the meniscus are comprised of very thin collagen fibrils laid down in a random manner. The collagen fibers of the interior are thicker and are arranged in a circumferential direction; smaller collagen fibrils branch off from these main collagen fiber bundles providing structural stability to this collection of fiber bundles (Slide V,23, left).

Slide V,23, right, shows the dependence of the tensile stress-strain behavior of circumferentially oriented surface-zone and deep-zone specimens and radially oriented surface-zone and deep-zone specimens. Clearly, the tensile modulus and strength of specimens parallel to the collagen fiber direction are much greater than those perpendicular to the collagen fiber direction. Surface-zone specimens do not show a statistically significant difference with respect to these two directions.

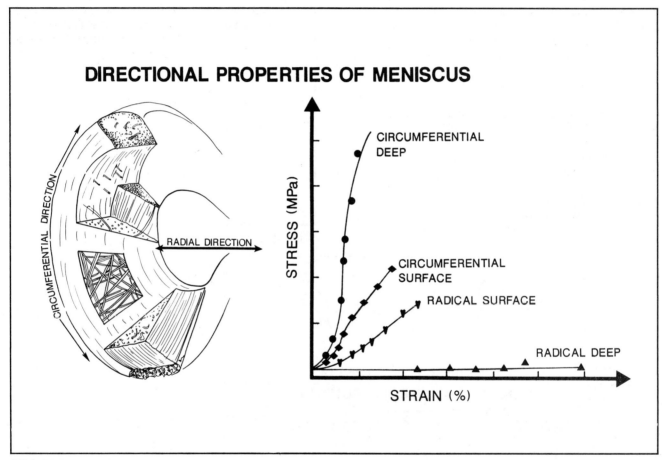

Slide V,23

Intervertebral Disc: Viscoelastic Creep

Biological structures and materials, especially soft tissues, often exhibit time-dependent stress-strain behaviors. Slide V,24 shows the creep response of an intervertebral disc. After an external load is applied, the deformation of the disc continues to increase until equilibrium is reached (lower right figure). The creep in the disc is largely due to the reorientation of the collagen fibrous network within the anulus of the disc and the redistribution of fluid within the nucleus pulposus. The rate of creep and the value of the final displacement are two specific deformational qualities characterizing the disc.

Intervertebral Disc: Viscoelastic Stress Relaxation

The viscoelastic behavior of the disc may also be expressed by a phenomenon known as "stress relaxation." Slide V,25 (middle) shows the stress response of an intervertebral disc to a constant compressive strain. After the strain is imposed, the stress required to maintain the strain continues to decrease, until equilibrium is reached. The same mechanisms responsible for creep, i.e., collagen network reorientation in the anulus and redistribution of fluids within the nucleus polposus, are responsible for stress relaxation. The rate of stress relaxation and the value of the final stress are two specific deformational qualities characterizing the disc. The final stress is inversely related to the final displacement, as measured in the creep experiment.

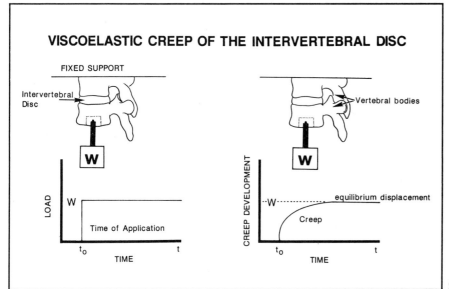

Slide V,24

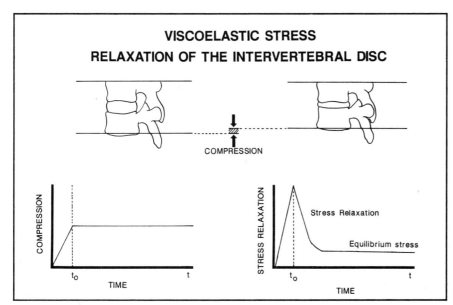

Slide V,25

Cartilage And Meniscus: Flow-Dependent Creep

The compressive viscoelastic creep (and stress relaxation) of highly hydrated soft tissues such as articular cartilage (approximately 80% water) and meniscus (approximately 73% water) is due to extrusion of the fluid from the tissue during compression. The upper left side of Slide V,26 depicts the fluid exudation process during a one-dimensional compression test. The upper right side of Slide V,26 shows the flow-dependent viscoelastic creep in compression caused by this fluid exudation process. The rate of fluid loss and hence creep are controlled by the permeability of the tissue. The value of the displacement at equilibrium and the rate of creep, as determined in the manner above, are used to define the compressive modulus at equilibrium and the permeability of tissues such as articular cartilage and meniscus.

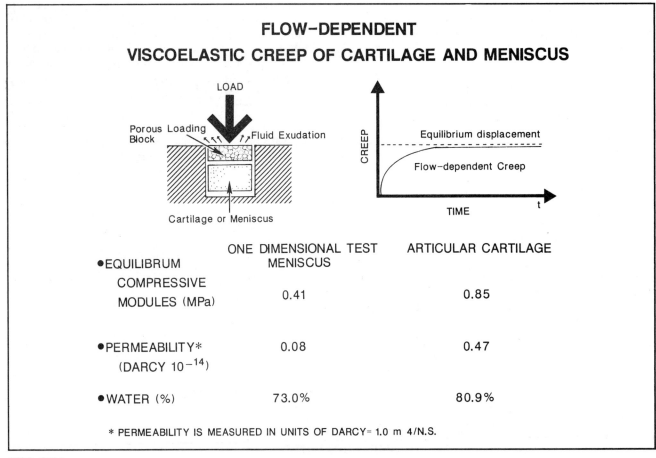

Slide V,26

Biomechanics of Structures: Musculoskeletal Organs

The biomechanical behavior of musculoskeletal tissues depends not only on the material properties of the tissues but on their structural properties as well. These structural properties are related to the various shapes and sizes of the organs in which the tissues are found. The amount and the orientation of loads experienced by these tissues differ according to body part. Thus, such factors as shape, and amount and orientation of load play an important role in distinguishing the structural properties of musculoskeletal tissues from their material properties.

Ligaments: Material vs. Structural Properties

Soft tissues provide an example of the differences between material and structural properties. At the microscopic level, ligaments are formed from collagen fibrils that combine to form collagen fibers and then fiber bundles. These bundles in turn are organized into a whole ligament with a given cross-sectional area and length. The mechanical behavior of the whole ligament depends on both the material properties of the

collagen and on the geometric arrangement of the fiber bundles (area and length). Since both material and geometry are involved, these are referred to as structural properties. Slide V,27 compares the breaking force of two ligaments by displaying tensile force-elongation curves for two ligaments of equal length. The one with a larger area fails at a greater force. The resistance of the ligament to elongation is given by the slope of the force-deformation curve and is referred to as the "stiffness." The ligament with a larger area also exhibits greater stiffness. Since both ligaments are made of the same material and are of the same length, the total elongation to failure is the same.

Slide V,28 provides similar comparisons between ligaments of equal cross-sectional area but different lengths. The longer ligament fails at a larger elongation. Although the fibers (the collagenous material) fail at the same percent elongation (strain), the longer ligament provides a greater total elongation. Note also that the stiffness (as measured by the slope of the load elongation curve) is less for the longer ligament, since it stretches further under the same force. Finally, since both ligaments have the same cross-sectional area, the failure load breaking strength multiplied by cross-sectional area for the two ligaments is the same.

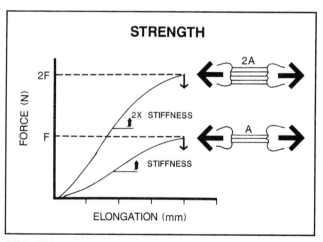

Slide V,27

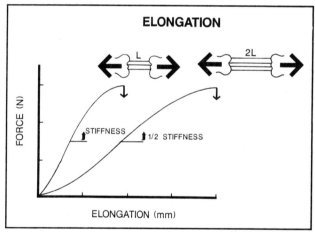

Slide V,28

Bending of Long Bones

Bones of the appendicular skeleton are long, slender, slightly curved elements that are loaded primarily by compressive forces applied at the joints. Slide V,29 shows the femur loaded by compressive forces applied at the hip and knee. Because of this curvature, bones are subjected *in vivo* to a combination of longitudinal axial compression and bending. To visualize bending, imagine grasping a yardstick and applying forces close to its ends such that it is flexed into a bowed shape. The amount of bowing depends on whether the yardstick is flexed in a vertical or a horizontal orientation. For the femur, the combination of compression and bending results in elongation of the convex surface and shortening of the concave surface. The stresses associated with the bending of curved members are also shown in Slide V,29. On the convex surface, tensile stresses are created. On the concave surface, the stresses are compressive. The relative magnitudes of the tensile and compressive stresses depend on a number of factors including the curvature of the bone and the magnitude of the longitudinal force.

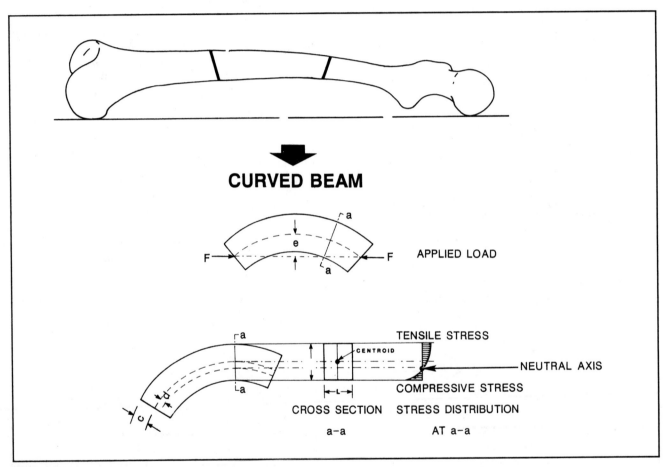

Slide V,29

Femoral Neck: Combined Compression and Bending

The femoral neck provides another example of combined loading. Slide V,30 shows a force acting on the femoral head as the combined result of a compressive force directed axially along the femoral neck and a transverse force directed perpendicular to the femoral neck. The axial compressive force results in the creation of compressive stresses at the mid-cervical cross-section. The transverse force results in bending stresses. These bending stresses are associated with tensile stresses on the superior surface of the femoral neck and compressive stresses on the inferior surface. When these two loading cases are combined, the tensile and compressive stresses on the superior neck tend to cancel and the compressive stresses on the inferior neck tend to sum. The result is a state of near zero stress on the superior surface of the neck and high compressive stresses on the inferior surface. The validity of this loading arrangement is substantiated by the pronounced thickness of the cervical cortex inferiorly (nearly 4 mm on average), as compared to the extremely thin cortex (.2-.4 mm) on the superior surface of the neck.

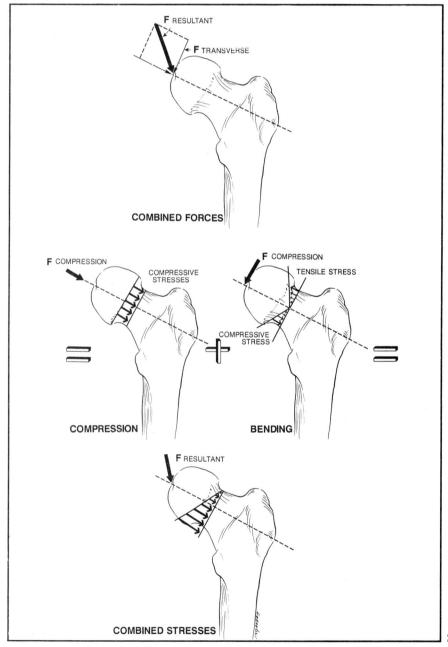

Slide V,30

Tibia: Torsion

Another important loading mode for long bones results from twisting (applying a moment) about the long axis of the bone. Slide V,31 shows a tibia subjected to torsion (as would occur in a twisting fall when skiing). Also shown are the internal shear stresses that occur on two typical cross-sections at the proximal and distal thirds. Note that the proximal third cross-section is of greater average radius and lower average thickness than the distal third, and yet the shear stresses in the proximal third are less. Torsional fractures of the tibia are more common in the distal third where the shear stresses are greatest. The above suggests that the shape and distribution of the cross-sectional area (in this case with respect to the long axis of the bone) significantly influence bone strength and rigidity.

Cross-Sectional Shapes: Area Moment of Inertia

The importance of a structure's geometric configuration to its rigidity and strength relates to the distribution of the structure's cross-sectional area with respect to an applied load. The geometric parameter that describes this area is called the area moment of inertia (sometimes referred to as the moment of inertia of a cross-section). Area moments of inertia for a number of representative cross-sectional shapes (solid cylinder, tube, rectangular bar and I-beam) are shown in Slide V,32. Area moments of inertia (written as I_{xx}) are expressed relative to neutral axes (x-x). In Slide V,32, these axes are shown as horizontal dotted lines on each cross-section. The neutral axis is defined as the central axis through the cross-section where the tensile stresses change to compression and bending is zero.

Bending Rigidity and Strength

To understand the rigidity and strength of any structure in response to loading, it is necessary to know 1) the mechanical properties of the material (Young's modulus, yield strength, ultimate strength); 2) the dimensions (thickness, width, length) and geometric configuration of the structure (cylinder, tube, rectangular bar); 3) the type of load (longitudinal, tension or compression, torsion, bending); and 4) the orientation of the structure with respect to the load. To demonstrate the influence of the orientation of the load on the bending rigidity of a structure, the following example is provided.

Slide V,33 (top) shows a wooden meter stick subjected to three-point bending applied first with the meter stick flat and then with the meter stick on edge. When it is flat, the meter stick bends easily; when on edge, almost no bending deflection occurs. In both cases, the bending forces and the material properties of the meter stick are the same, and yet, when on edge, the meter stick can resist bending deflection (i.e., its bending rigidity has increased greatly). This increase in bending rigidity is determined by the two different orientations of the meter stick with respect to the applied bending loads.

As the bending forces increase, the flat meter stick fails, while the meter stick on edge remains intact. (Note that failure has occurred because the bending stresses on the top and bottom surfaces of the meter stick have exceeded the tensile or compressive strength of the wood.) The bending stresses are also influenced by the distance

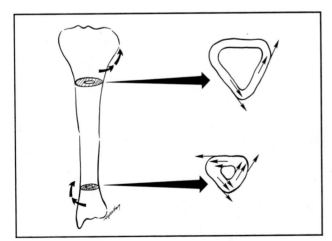

Slide V,31

CROSS-SECTION	MOMENT OF INERTIA
x – ⊙ – x (radius r)	$I_{xx} = \pi r^4 / 4$
x – ⊙ – x (radii r_o, r_i)	$I_{xx} = \pi(r_o^4 - r_i^4)/4$
rectangle, width w, depth d	$I_{xx} = w d^3 / 12$
I-beam, width w, depth d, flange a	$I_{xx} = \dfrac{w d^3 - (w-a)(d-2a)^3}{12}$

Slide V,32

(c) from the neutral axis of the top and bottom surfaces. The bending strength is directly proportional to c and inversely proportional to I_{xx}:bending strength $\sim C/I_{xx}$. For the rectangular cross-section shown in Slide V,32, the distance c is d/2.

Given the example of bending the meter stick, the role of the orientation of the cross-section can now be described more precisely. With the meter stick flat, most of its cross-sectional area is close to the neutral axis and the structure bends easily. With the meter stick on edge, more of the material is distributed at a greater distance from the neutral axis and the bending rigidity is great. In quantitative terms, the bending deflection is inversely proportional to the area moment of inertia:bending deflection $\sim 1/I_{xx}$. By interchanging roles for the width (w) and the depth (d) of the rectangular cross-section and by assuming that w = d/4, it can be easily demonstrated that the bending deflection of the flat meter stick should be 16 times the deflection of the meter stick on edge. This evidence points to the importance of cross-sectional orientation on the bending rigidity of a struc-

ture. These factors also help explain why the I-beam shown in Slide V, 32 is such an efficient cross-sectional shape. The I-beam is loaded in the same way as the meter stick on edge; most of the cross-sectional material is distributed at a maximum distance from the neutral axis where it contributes most to the bending rigidity and strength.

Bones, unlike the meter stick or the I-beam, are subjected to bending loads in many directions. In addition, as with the tibia, long bones are subjected to torsional moments about the long axis. For these loading conditions, the most efficient shape is a circle cylinder because it provides an equivalent area moment about any transverse axis. However, as with the meter stick and I-beam, the material of the cylinder most efficient for resisting bending or torsion is located at the greatest distance from the transverse or longitudinal axes, respectively. For this reason, as well as for the obvious advantage of storing marrow and establishing a medullary blood supply, long bones have evolved cross-sectional geometries that are generally tubular.

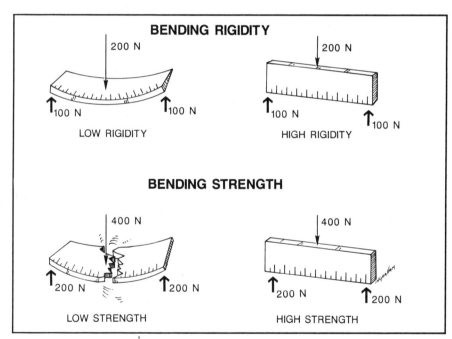

Slide V,33

Effect of Aging on Bending Rigidity

Slide V,34 demonstrates that a cylindrical tube more efficiently resists bending than does a solid cylinder of the same cross-sectional area. Three cylindrical rods are shown. Bar A is a solid cylinder with a radius of .94 cm. Bar B is a hollow tube of outer radius 1.09 cm and inner radius .53 cm. Bar C is also a hollow tube, but the outer radius and the inner radius have been increased over bar B by 1.25 cm and .76 cm, respectively. The values for the cross-sectional areas and moments of inertia of these simple shapes are also shown. Since the tensile or compressive strengths are inversely proportional to the cross-sectional area ($\sigma = -F/A$), bars A and B exhibit similar strengths and bar C is increased in strength by about 3%. In bending loading, however, the more favorable distribution of the cross-sectional area results in increases in bending strengths by factors of 1.49 and 1.93 for bars B and C. In particular, the changes in inner and outer radii for tube C in comparison to B result in an increase in bending strength by a factor of about 1.29. These idealized cross-sections are based on the approximate dimensions of the human femoral mid-shaft and on the known changes in cross-sectional properties that occur with age. These results indicate that in human long bones, although the cortical thickness of bone decreases with age, a compensatory remodeling of the cross-sectional geometry occurs so that the bone's structural properties are maintained.

If these concepts are applied to the solid cylinder in Slide V,32, the moment of inertia is proportional to the fourth power of the radius. Since bending rigidity is the deflection per unit bending load, the bending rigidity of a circular cylinder increases as the fourth power of the radius. As with the meter stick, the bending strength increases with the third power of the radius (since the distance to surface of the bar is r/2). Although bending rigidity and strength have been emphasized here, it is important to note that similar concepts apply to the torsional rigidity and strength. In torsion, however, the cross-sectional parameter that describes the resistance to torsion is called polar moment of inertia, J, and is expressed with respect to the long axis of the cylinder. The polar moment of inertia, J, of a solid cylinder is equal to $\pi r4/2$. Thus, as with bending, the resistance to twist (the torsional rigidity) increases with the fourth power of the radius. The torsional strength varies as the third power of the radius. These factors help explain the differences in fracture incidence (noted in Slide V,31) for the proximal and distal third of the tibia. As shown in the slide, the proximal cross-section places more of the available material at a greater distance from the longitudinal axis. Therefore, the polar moment of inertia and the torsional strength of the proximal cross-section is greater, and fractures tend to occur at the distal third (despite the increased cortical thickness at that site).

This section has focused on the differences between material behavior (at the tissue level) and structural behavior (at the whole bone or joint level). The biomechanical behavior of a structure results from the combination of material properties and the geometric configuration of the structure with respect to the applied load. In simple tension or compression the cross-sectional area influences the axial rigidity and strength. In bending and torsion, the area and polar moments of inertia control the structural response. Relatively subtle changes in these geometric parameters can result in large changes in the rigidity and strength of the whole bone.

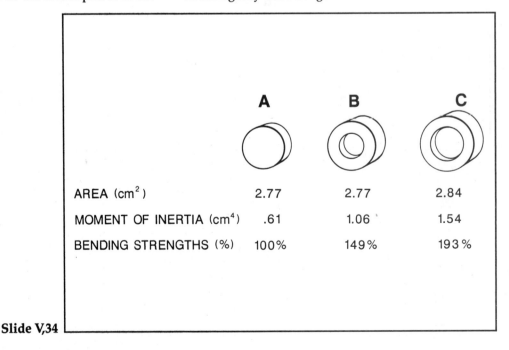

	A	B	C
AREA (cm^2)	2.77	2.77	2.84
MOMENT OF INERTIA (cm^4)	.61	1.06	1.54
BENDING STRENGTHS (%)	100%	149%	193%

Slide V,34

Tibial Plateau: Load Transmission

During daily activities, such as level walking and stair climbing, the loads acting on the joint surfaces may be as high as ten times body weight, see Slides V,5-V,9). Slide V,35 shows a pair of forces acting on the knee joint. The transmission of these forces from one articulating surface onto the other is a complex process. Also shown are the compressive stress patterns acting over the meniscal-tibial plateau at 0°, 15° and 30° flexion. The salient features of these compressive stress patterns are that (1) most of the compressive stress acts over the meniscal surface; (2) the compressive stress pattern depends on the flexion angle; and (3) very high compressive stresses exist at the meniscal-tibial plateau surface.

Cartilage-Cartilage Friction: Static and Dynamic

The coefficient of friction (μ) is defined as the ratio of the magnitudes of two forces: $\mu = T/N$, where T is the transverse force required to slide one surface over another and N is the normal force used to press the two surfaces together, (see inset Slide V,36). The coefficient of friction for a well lubricated stainless steel bearing is about 0.03 and for skating on ice is 0.02. For a 750 n person (150 lb) skating on one skate, it takes 15 n (3 lb) of force to overcome the frictional resistance between the ice and skate. The frictional resistance for cartilage-to-cartilage contact with synovial fluid is shown in Slide V,36. Under dynamic (oscillating) compressive loads, the coefficient of friction remains very low up to 2.0 MN/mxm (300 psi). Under static (constant) compressive loads, the coefficient of friction initially decreases and then dramatically increases with increasing load.

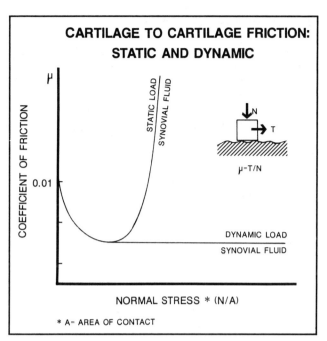

Slide V,36

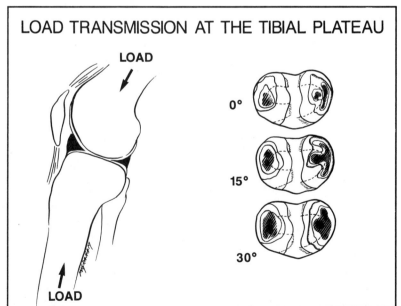

Slide V,35

Joint Lubrication: Fluid-Film Generation

One mechanism responsible for the remarkably low coefficient of friction for cartilage sliding or rolling over cartilage is fluid-film lubrication. In diarthrodial joints, the liquid lubricant comes from two sources: (1) synovial fluid; and (2) articular cartilage. Under static loads, as shown in Slide V,36 the coefficient of friction is very low, although it does increase dramatically with increasing normal force. This low frictional value is due to the lubrication effect rendered by a thin layer of synovial fluid. Under dynamic loading conditions, the low coef- ficient of friction is due to the lubricant film created from the cartilage exudate released by the mechanical pumping action of the oscillating load or the action of a moving load. Slide V,37 shows the mechanical pumping action as one joint surface rolls or slides over the other; fluid is forced out at the leading edge of the contact area and reabsorbed at the trailing edge. The arrows at the upper right of the slide show the flow paths by which the exudation/imbibition process occurs. The high and low pressure regions and the leading and trailing edges of the load-bearing contact area are shown at the bottom right of the slide.

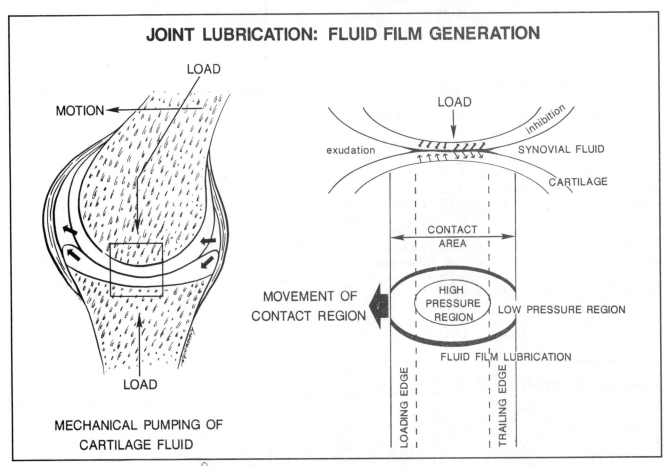

Slide V,37

Coeff friction = $\dfrac{\text{frictional resistance}}{\text{load}}$

Cartilage: Rate of Wear

Friction and lubrication between two moving surfaces are intrinsically related to wear. In general, friction causes wear and lubrication prevents wear. There are two types of lubrication: 1) boundary lubrication; and 2) fluid-film lubrication. Boundary lubrication prevents wear by means of the monolayer of lubricating glycoprotein found in the synovial fluid adsorbed onto the articular surface. Fluid-flim lubrication is the most effec-

tive method of preventing wear. Both synovial fluid and cartilage exudate provide the fluid required for fluid-film lubrication. Cartilage exudate is most effective in maintaining a very low value for the coefficient of friction. Slide V,38 shows the wear rate of cartilage under three experimental conditions: (1) cartilage against cartilage with synovial fluid; (2) cartilage against cartilage with buffer only; and (3) cartilage against a stainless steel surface with a fluid buffer. Note the high wear of cartilage against stainless steel.

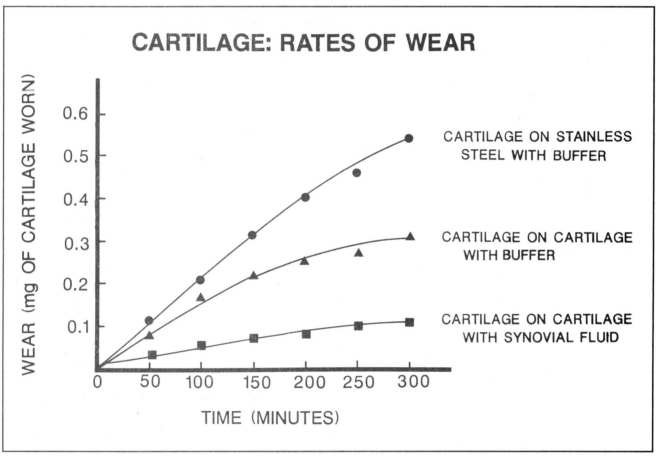

Slide V,38

Articular Cartilage: Compressive Stresses

Because cartilage is a two-phase material (80% water and 20% organic solid), the state of stress in cartilage is controlled by the rate at which fluid moves through the tissue (internal tissue permeability) and compressive modulus of the tissue at equilibrium. (Slide V,39) Thus, the state of stress acting in cartilage is very complex. Stresses of all types exist: tension, compression and shear. Slide V,39 bottom shows the regions where maximum tensile, compressive and shear stresses exist within a layer of cartilage when the joint is compressed. Surface fibrillations are due to the high tensile stresses running parallel to the surface within the contact region. The surface zone of normal articular cartilage has more collagen and is stiffer compared to the deeper zones. The collagen resists the large tensile stresses developed during joint loading. Damage to cartilage in the deep zones results from the high shear stresses acting along and near the tidemark directly under the contact area.

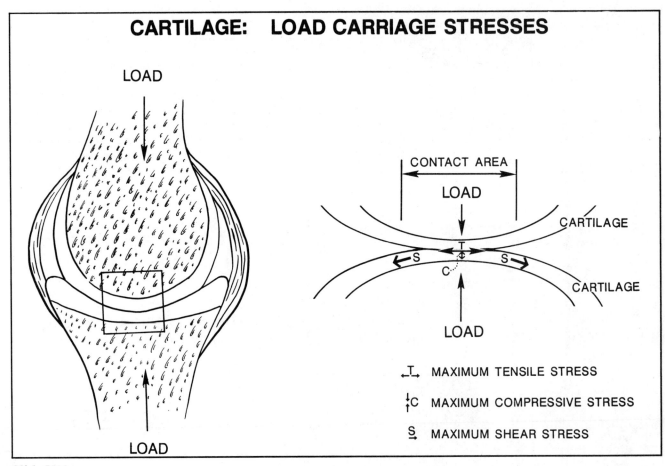

Slide V,39

Muscle: Mechanical Behavior

Slide V,40 illustrates the two ways in which muscle generates forces: the resistance of the natural material to being stretched (passive force); and voluntary muscle contraction. The latter can be assumed to be a structural property of muscle that changes with the degree of neurological activation to the muscle. The most probable passive load deformation curve (curve 1) appears similar to the toe and linear regions of the load deformation curves of other soft tissues. The length of the muscle at the point where this force begins is termed the muscle's "resting length." The voluntary tension curve (curve 3) is produced by active muscle contraction. The muscle can generate a force by active muscle contraction even when it is shorter than its "resting length." The total tension curve (curve 2) developed in a muscle is the sum of the active muscle contraction (curve 3) and the muscle's passive force (curve 1). For the same degree of muscle stimulation, the amount of voluntary tension produced by a muscle is dependent but not proportional to its length. The maximum voluntary force produced by a muscle occurs at its "resting length." If the muscle is stretched beyond the "resting length" the "active

force" decreases dramatically. The net total muscle force (curve 2) does not decrease to the same degree owing to the contribution of the passive force required to stretch the muscle beyond its "resting length," (curve 1). The fall-off in the voluntary force beyond the resting length occurs because the actin-myosin molecule bonds producing the active force become physically disassociated at this point.

The force developed within a muscle is dependent upon many factors: the number of motor units within the muscle that are recruited; the number of recruitment stimuli per unit time to a given motor unit; the inherent nature of the muscle itself, i.e., the number of slow-and fast-twitch fibers within the muscle; and the manner in which the muscle changes its length. Slide V,40 illustrates how the manner in which change in length contributes to the force of muscle contraction. In an isometric contraction, the length of the muscle does not change; the force is increased by increasing the recruitment frequency. In an eccentric contraction, the muscle lengthens, and force increase depends on both the number of motor units recruited and the rapidity of their recruitment.

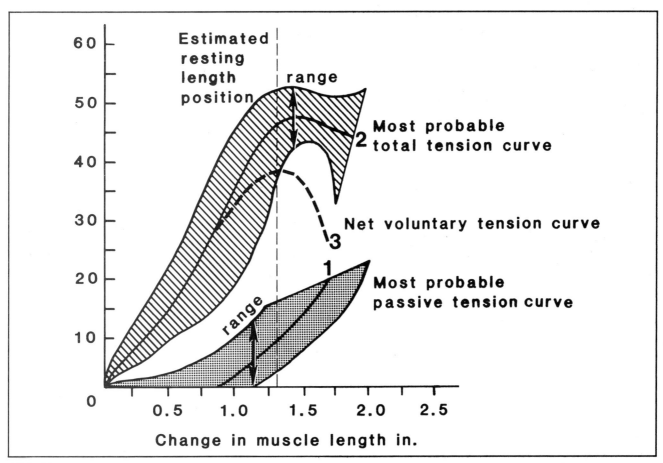

Slide V,40

Muscles develop these forces to perform work or to absorb energy. Slide V,41, bottom left side, illustrates that when the quadriceps performs work, it shortens and accelerates the limb. The bottom right side of Slide V,41 illustrates that when the muscle absorbs energy it lengthens, decelerating the body and absorbing force. In an isometric contraction, such as standing on one limb (bottom middle slide), muscle length does not change and no work is done.

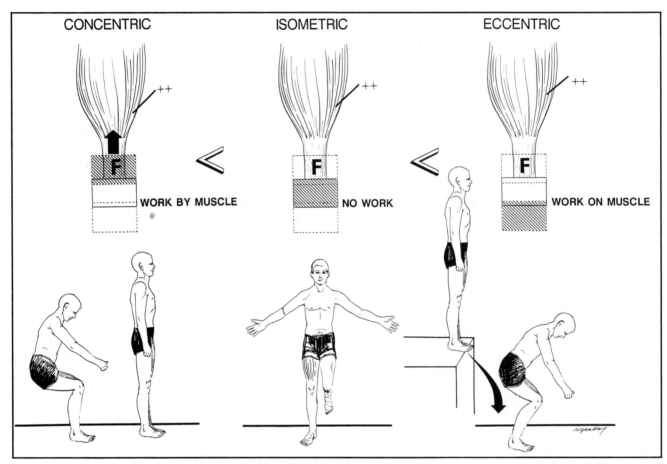

Slide V,41

Biomechanics of Pathological Processes

In the previous three sections, basic concepts in biomechanics have been presented in relation to the material and structural properties of the musculoskeletal system. This section discusses pathological processes of the musculoskeletal system and how they alter the biomechanical behavior of its tissues and organs. This altered behavior, in turn, affects the pathological processes.

Chondromalacia Patellae: Contact Pressures

Joint abnormalities such as chondromalacia and osteoarthritis alter the manner of load transmission from one articulating surface to the other. Slide V,42 illustrates the three forces acting on the patella to maintain static equilbrium. The force acting on the patellar surface results from the action/reaction contact between the patella and the femoral groove during articulation. This force is distributed over the patellar surface as a compressive stress. The pattern of distribution of this compressive stress differs depending on the biomechanical quality of the articular cartilage. The center of Slide V,42 shows a typical pattern of stress distribution for normal patellar cartilage. On the right is shown the pattern of stress distribution on the surface of a patella with chrondromalacia. Loading conditions were similar for both patellae. The stress distribution differences result from differences in the material properties of the cartilage from the two patellae.

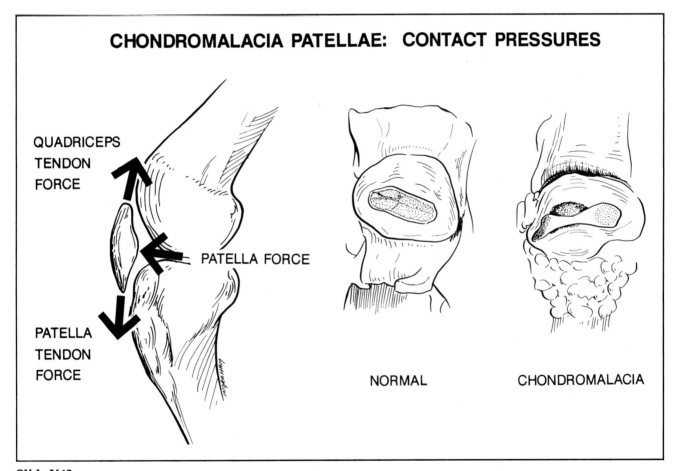

CHONDROMALACIA PATELLAE: CONTACT PRESSURES

QUADRICEPS TENDON FORCE

PATELLA FORCE

PATELLA TENDON FORCE

NORMAL

CHONDROMALACIA

Slide V,42

Osteoarthritis: Material Property Changes of Articular Cartilage with Change in Composition

Osteoarthritis is primarily an articular cartilage disease. Slide V,43 shows the changes in the compressive modulus and shear modulus of articular cartilage with changes in proteoglycan (uronic acid) and collagen composition. Collagen and proteoglycans are the main load-carrying structural molecules of soft connective tissues such as articular cartilage, tendons, and ligaments. Normal stress distribution and lubrication depend on normal biomechanical properties of collagen and proteoglycans, which are maintained by the chondrocytes. Slide V,43 clearly demonstrates how cartilage is weakened by changes in concentrations of collagen and proteoglycans.

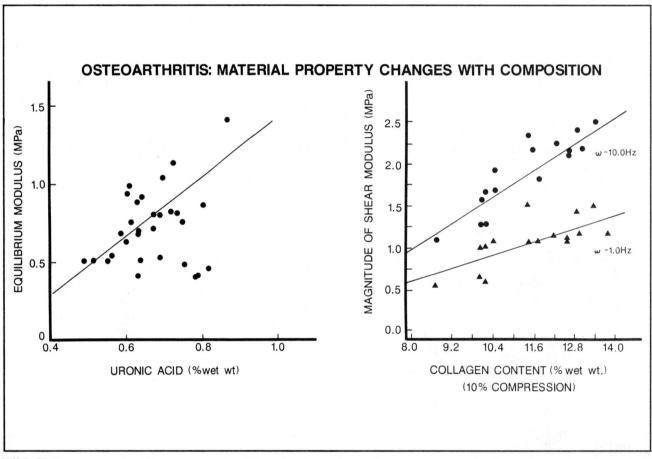

Slide V,43

Osteoarthritis: Material Property Changes of Articular Cartilage with Water Content

In osteoarthritis, the earliest change of cartilage composition is increased hydration, or water content, as shown in Slide V,44. This change is caused by a number of factors: (1) weakening of the collagen network due to fibrillation; (2) disorganization of the proteoglycan molecular structure; (3) loss of the fragmented proteoglycans by diffusion; and 4) loss of the collagen fibrils by wear. The weakened collagen network permits increased swelling and the loss of proteoglycans allows more space in the interstitium for water. An increased water content would increase cartilage porosity and decrease cartilage density. These changes have profound effects on cartilage permeability (left side of slide) and cartilage compressive compliance, defined as the reciprocal of the equilibrium compressive modulus (right side of slide). Large increases in tissue permeability with osteoarthrits result in poor fluid-film generation for lubrication, and large increases in the compressive compliance with osteoarthritis alter normal load-carriage mechanisms. Both processes accelerate the wear and further breakdown of articular cartilage.

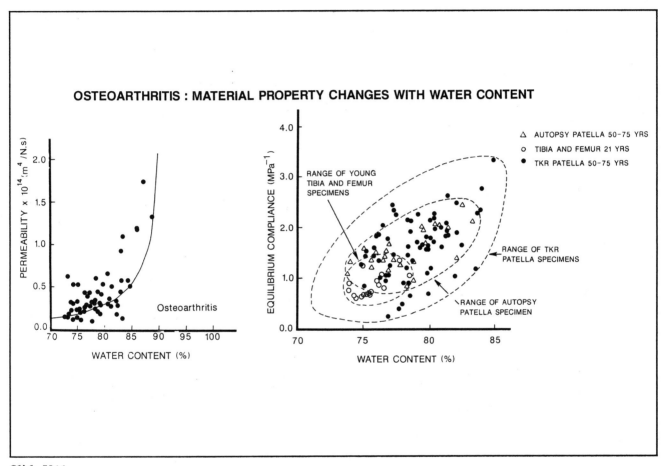

Slide V,44

Joint Stiffness: Effects of Immobilization

The effects of reduced stress on bone are well known, as are the effects of immobilization in producing the atrophy of muscle mass. The effects of immobilization on fibrous connective tissues are more difficult to measure. Contractures are commonly observed following prolonged immobilization of musculoskeletal injuries. Experimental studies have shown that forces required to flex and extend immobilized knees are considerably higher than forces required to flex and extend normal knees (Slide V,45). The lower left of Slide V,45 shows that as a normal knee is extended and then flexed, the torque, or force, remains low and constant. In a knee that has been immobilized (lower right, Slide V,45), the torque increases as the knee is extended. When the knee is then flexed, the torque at the beginning of the motion is greater than at the end. The difference between the amount of effort required to extend and then flex the knee (the area inside the loop in the slide) reflects the amount of energy needed to move the joint and overcome the stiffness of the knee. Such increases in knee-

joint stiffness can be attributed to a number of changes in the joint's periarticular connective tissues, including adhesions, pannus formation, capsular contractures and ligament shortenings.

Bone-Ligament Complex: Effects of Immobilization and Remobilization

The effects of immobilization on the mechanical properties of a bone-ligament-bone complex are also very significant (Slide V,46). After nine weeks of immobilization, the maximum force, and the energy-absorbing ability (area underneath the load-deformation curve) of a rabbit medial collateral ligament (MCL) are reduced by approximately one-third when compared to the contralateral nonimmobilized control. Immobilization significantly weakens the ligament-bone junction. As a result, the failure mode of the bone-ligament structure in the immobilized knee is usually by avulsion. Immobilization has a significant deleterious effect on both the ligament substance and the ligament-bone junction.

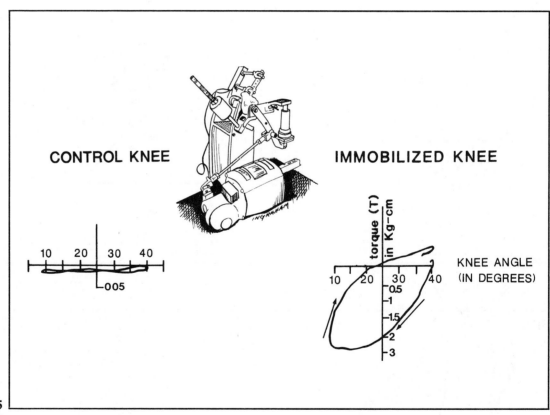

Slide V,45

Experimental studies have shown that the tensile properties of the rabbit MCL-bone structure continue to be inferior with nine weeks of remobilization (cage activities) following nine weeks of immobilization. The mechanical properties of the MCL substance appear to recover quickly and completely, while the bone-ligament junction does not. Slide V,47 shows that the load-deformation curve of the MCL substance of an experimental knee becomes almost identical to that of the control knee at ligament strain up to 5%. Studies have also shown that a year of daily conditioning is required to recover the strength and failure mode of the primate's femur-ACL-bone structure following eight weeks of immobilization. It is important to recognize that there are asynchronous recovery rates among various tissues in the bone-ligament structure.

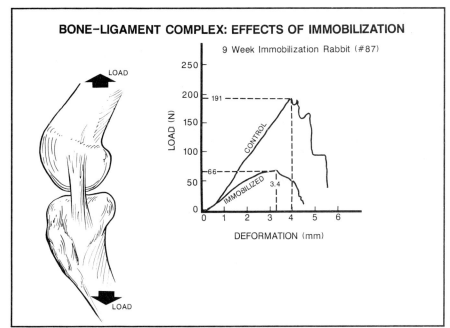

BONE–LIGAMENT COMPLEX: EFFECTS OF IMMOBILIZATION

9 Week Immobilization Rabbit (#87)

Slide V,46

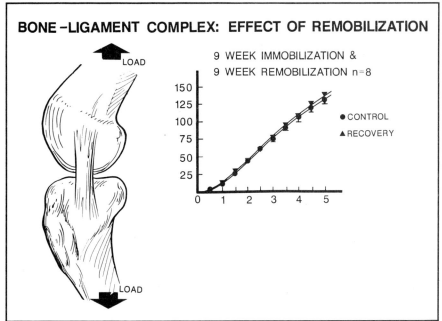

BONE –LIGAMENT COMPLEX: EFFECT OF REMOBILIZATION

9 WEEK IMMOBILIZATION &
9 WEEK REMOBILIZATION n=8

● CONTROL
▲ RECOVERY

Slide V,47

Pathomechanics of Spinal Osteoporosis

Osteoporosis is a skeletal condition characterized by a reduction in bone volume and an increased vulnerability to fracture, particularly of the femoral neck and vertebra. The prevalence of osteoporosis is well recognized, with 50% of women 45 years old or older exhibiting radiographic evidence of osteoporosis of the lumbar spine. While basic research on osteoporosis has focused primarily on cellular and metabolic mechanisms, it is bone fracture that represents the overriding clinical consequence of the disease, with an estimated four million people in the United States having osteoporosis severe enough to result in vertebral fracture. Slide V,48 shows a fracture of the lumbar spine in a 58-year-old woman with osteoporosis. Since many of the treatment modalities for osteoporosis are themselves associated with some risk, it is important to develop noninvasive methods to assess fracture risk in individual patients.

Quantitative computed tomography (QCT), as shown in Slide V,49, can be used to provide clinical assessments of fracture risk. Note that the QCT scan provides information on both the vertebral geometry and on the trabecular density. Based on the density-strength relationships described in Slide V,17, such scans could be used to provide individual assessments of lumbar fracture risk. Slide V,49 also shows the correlation between *in vitro* QCT scans of cadaveric lumbar spines and subsequent direct measurements of small cylindrical specimens of vertebral trabecular bone. As shown, the correlation between QCT number (in Hounsfield units) and apparent density is very strong ($R^2 = 0.89$, $p > 0.0001$). This suggests that this relationship can be used as the basis for a noninvasive prediction of vertebral strength. According to the density-compressive strength relationships presented earlier, the vertebral compressive strength should be related to the square of the apparent density.

Slide V,50 shows a log-log plot of vertebral compressive strength (failure load/area) versus the trabecular apparent densities. A best-fit power log curve, shown as the solid line, has an exponent of 2.26 and an $R^2 = 0.82$ ($p > 0.0001$). This exponent does not differ significantly from the squared relationship shown as a broken line that is the expected finding shown in Slide V,17. This result confirms that the squared relationships between vertebral compressive strength and density not only can be used to determine local material properties but also to make assessments of the structural properties of whole regions such as the vertebral body.

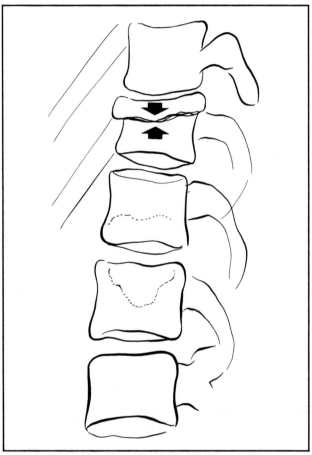

Slide V,48

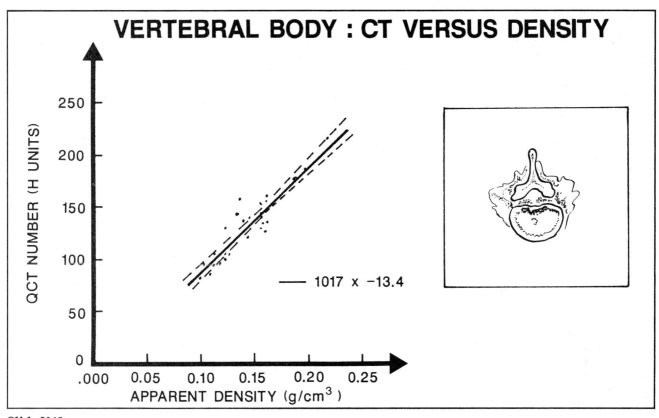

Slide V,49

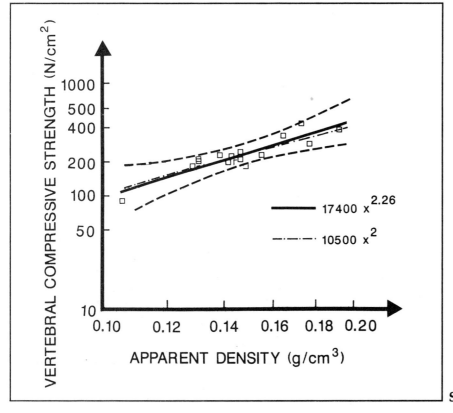

Slide V,50

Stress Concentration: Effects Caused by Metastatic Defects in Diaphysis

Slide V,51 shows a metastatic defect in the mid-femoral diaphysis of a 53-year-old woman with breast cancer. In many instances it is preferable to stabilize such regions prior to the occurrence of a pathological fracture. It is then necessary to determine when the bone is sufficiently weakened by the defect to warrant internal fixation. In engineering, the presence of a local defect resulting in increased local stresses is referred to as a "stress concentration" because the stresses around the defect are greater than would be predicted from the loss in area associated with the defect. Similar stress concentrations occur in areas where screw holes have been placed, or cortical strut grafts have been removed. The stress concentrating effects of metastatic defects on long bones have received little attention. In fact, the most widely quoted criterion for prophylactic stabilization (the existence of a 1-inch diameter defect) does not take into account that stress concentrating effects must be described as ratios of the size of the defect to the size of the original structure. The stress concentrating effect of a 1-inch diameter defect would be different in bones of different diameters.

Slide V,52 shows the reduction in strength associated with an increase in the ratio of hole diameter to bone diameter (a/d_o). The loss of strength is most rapid as a/d_o increases to 0.2, at which point the bone has lost approximately 40% of its original strength. When a/d_o reaches 0.8, the bone strength is reduced to 30% of its normal value. These results indicate that the ratio of defect size to bone diameter is important. Many fac-

tors influence the decision to stabilize an impending pathological fracture. Nevertheless, the current recommendation that stabilization be done when the metastatic defect involves 50% of the cortex is probably not sufficiently stringent. At this point, the bone retains only 30% of its normal strength. In any case, it is important to measure the ratio of defect size to bone size in order to estimate to stress-concentrating effect of a metastatic defect in bone.

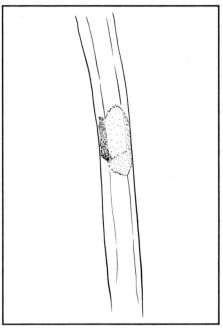

Slide V,51

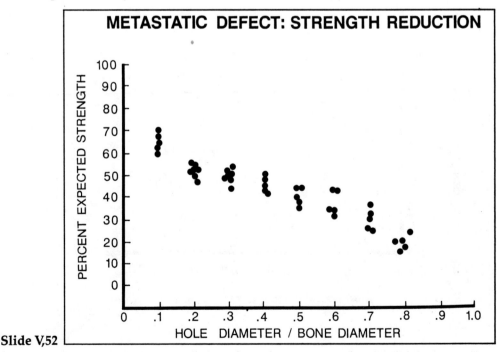

Slide V,52

Tendon-Muscle Junction: Effects of Atrophy

The biomechanical effects of tendon-muscle atrophy are illustrated in Slide V,53. The rupture of the Achilles tendon may be considered the soft tissue counterpart of the bony stress (fatigue) fracture. During normal activity, the gastroc/soleus muscle-tendon complex operates in an eccentric manner. Increased activity (such as playing tennis) somewhat increases the tensile force borne by this tissue, but more significantly increases the frequency of such tensile forces. Failure occurs because the tissue cannot repair itself quickly enough. Under such circumstances, it is rare for the rupture to occur in the muscle's substance, as increased motor recruitment is available to protect each fiber. It is in the tendinous portion of the complex that such ruptures occur.

Trendelenburg Gait: Physiological Compensation to Maintain Dynamic Moment Equilibrium

A variety of neuromuscular/skeletal disorders cause a decrease in the hip abductor muscle effort during the single-limb stance phase of normal gait. Such muscle weakness can occur secondary to nerve damage, disuse atrophy, or secondary to degenerative arthritis of the hip. We have seen from Slides V,5 and V,6 that the concept of equilibrium about any joint, whether conditions are of a dynamic (walking) or static (one-legged stance) nature, results in a large compressive joint reaction force. To lessen the pain arising within a degenerated joint, while allowing the patient to function, the abductor muscle force must be reduced. This tends to favor body weight, thereby rotating the pelvis clockwise. When the muscle is weak, the same phenomenon

occurs (Slide V,54). This moment must therefore be reduced. The moment can be reduced by moving the trunk laterally over the involved hip. The moment created by the body's weight can be further reduced during dynamic conditions by decreasing the body's acceleration (walking more slowly) and the amount of single-limb stance time.

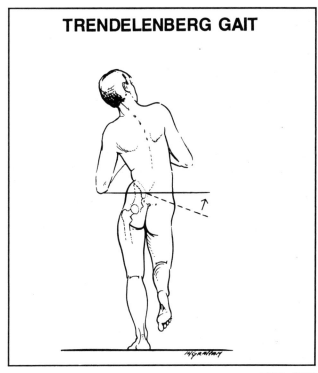

TRENDELENBERG GAIT

Slide V,54

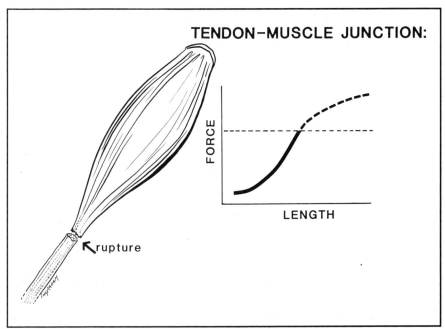

TENDON-MUSCLE JUNCTION:

FORCE

LENGTH

rupture

Slide V,53

Crouched Posture: Static Normal Equilibrium

In the typical crouched position, Slide V,55, the ankle is dorsiflexed and the knee and hip are flexed. In this position, the body weight's moment arm about each joint is significantly increased. Since the muscle moment arm is fixed at each joint, an increased muscle force must be produced to maintain an upright posture. Because these joints are flexed, each muscle produces its force at a length greater than its resting length, hence requiring recruitment of a greater number of motor units and more frequent stimulation of the recruited motor units.

Biomechanics of Musculoskeletal Treatment and Healing

Proximal Femoral Prosthesis: Bending Moment

When the proximal support of a femoral prosthetic component is insufficient, but the distal support is rigidly fixed, stress on the femoral stem may be increased three-fold. This increased stress could lead to plastic deformation or fatigue fracture (Slide V,56). Several other factors related to increasing the bending moment on the femur can also increase the chance of femoral stem "failure" or loosening. Since the bending moment is equal to the moment arm times the joint reaction force and the latter

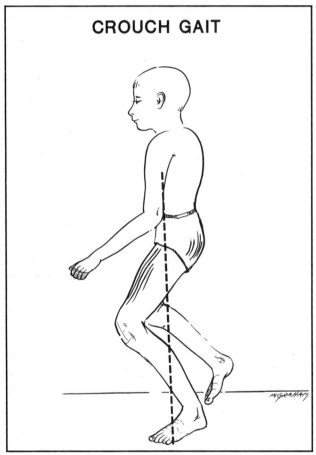

Slide V,55

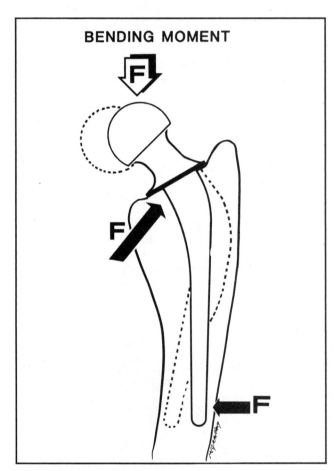

Slide V,56

is equal to 3-4 times the body weight, increases in body weight affect the bending moment. Additionally, since hip muscle forces are necesssary to accelerate and decelerate body weight, an increase in a person's walking speed or distance will increase the number of times and/or the size of moment applied to the prosthesis with shorter neck components. When the neck shaft angle is increased, such as in valgus placement, the bending moments may decrease. The increase in joint reaction force produced by an increased abductor force needed to offset the reduction in its level arm may negate the benefits of a short prosthetic neck or valgus placement.

Total Knee Replacement: Joint Instability

Joint stability is determined by the range of rotational and translational motions referenced to three perpendicular axes. At each joint, for each type of motion, the range of motion allowed differs. The range may be limited by bone or by ligament. At the knee joint, Slide V,57, stability is largely determined by ligamentous forces resisting anteroposterior and medial lateral translational forces, and varus/valgus and internal/external rotational moments. The articular surfaces provide resistance to compression and act as the fulcrum about which body

weight, flexor/extensor muscle forces, and ligamentous forces act to maintain equilibrium. With joint destruction, the fulcrum is altered; ligament length and resistive forces change; and the stress distribution in the articular cartilage in both compression and shear are altered.

As shown in Slide V,57, the changed mechanics provide decreased resistance to motion along or about the different knee axes: the joint is unstable. With time, these pathomechanics in themselves can lead to further joint destruction. To obtain optimal results from joint replacement arthroplasty, the proper selection of prostheses, the position of the prosthesis in the bone, and if necessary, the restoration of normal ligament length are all necessary. If normal mechanics and joint stability are not restored, prosthetic loosening or bone resorption could result.

Muscle Tendon Transfer: Effect of Force Versus Moment Arm Reduction

A variety of surgical procedures have been described to alter the magnitude of the moment produced by a muscle about a given joint; the force magnitude and/or the moment arm must change. If a muscle does not have the potential to develop an adequate force, it is difficult to increase the moment arm enough to allow the muscle to compensate for it. The transfer of the anterior tibialis muscle posteriorly to the calcaneus cannot adequately substitute for a weak gastroc/soleus muscle. In contrast, the torque produced by the spasticity of the gastroc/soleus muscles can be reduced in a variety of ways. By lengthening the Achilles tendon, the muscle force can be reduced without changing the moment arm. Alternatively, as shown in Slide V,58, the insertion of the muscle can be placed closer to the ankle's axes, reducing the moment arm. As the change to the muscle-tendon length is minimal, little alteration results in the manner by which the muscle behaves.

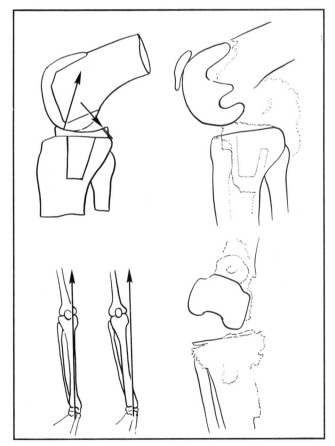

Slide V,57

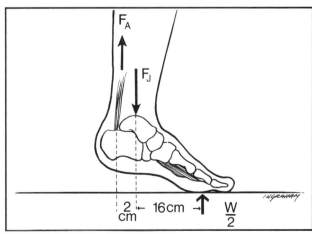

Slide V,58

Fracture Healing: Callus vs. Osteonal Union

Interfragmentary relative motion at a fracture site influences the morphologic and radiologic pattern of fracture healing. Slide V,59 demonstrates fractures of both bones of the forearm, with the fracture of the radius fixed by a compression plate and the fracture of the ulna healing without fixation. Two markedly different healing patterns are observed: the ulna displays a pronounced callus and the plated fracture very little evidence of callus formation. Healing of the plated fracture is proceeding by "osteonal union," i.e., by direct cortical reconstruction without the intervention of a bridging callus. This mode of fracture healing has also been referred to as "primary bone healing" and is presumed to be related to the rigidity of fixation provided by the compression plate. In the unplated fracture, the fracture fragments must be stabilized through the development of a periosteal bridging callus before cortical reconstruction can occur. The latter process, which occurs with the use of cast fixation, has been referred to as "natural healing." It is important to note, however, that despite strong clincial views on the relative advantages of these two approaches to fracture treatment (cast versus plate fixation), little objective biomechanical evidence exists to suggest that either approach results in accelerated healing times or in stiffer or stronger fractures at earlier stages in the healing process.

Four Biomechanical Stages of Fracture Healing

Clinical classification schemes for staging the healing of a fracture are based primarily on radiographic criteria. Classification schemes based on objective biomechanical criteria would allow a more precise determination of the appropriate time for cast removal and the resumption of normal activities. Slide V,60 shows torque-deformation curves for healing rabbit osteotomies at various healing times (in days). Until about day 26, the healing osteotomies fail because of a rubbery, soft-tissue behavior characterized by low torque values and large angular deformations. About day 27, an abrupt increase in stiffness occurs. Thereafter, the stiffness (defined as the slope of the torque-deformation curve) remains approximately constant, but the failure torque continues to increase to a maximum value at day 56. Based on these torque-deformation curves and on the observed patterns of failure of the tested bones, we can classify fracture healing into four biomechanical stages: Stage 1—failure through the original fracture site with a low stiffness, rubbery pattern; Stage 2—failure through the fracture site with a high stiffness, hard tissue pattern; Stage 3—failure partially through the original fracture site with a high stiffness pattern; Stage 4—failure unrelated to the original fracture site with a high stiffness pattern. Presumably, similar fracture healing stages occur in patients, but these stages are only roughly correlated to the radiographic appearance of the fracture. One interesting clinical finding related to these results is the widely reported increase in fracture site rigidity, sometimes called "stickiness," that many patients describe relatively early in the course of healing.

Fracture Healing: Rigidity vs. Strength

The stiffness or rigidity of a healing fracture returns to normal at a rate much faster than does the strength. Slide V,61 shows a plot of strength ratio (strength of a healing experimental osteotomy divided by strength of the contralateral, untreated control) to a similarly defined stiffness ratio (fractured/intact). All data are from osteotomies tested after 5 weeks of healing. Although these data indicate that healing rates are widely variable, in a striking number of cases the stiffness ratio approaches normal almost exactly twice as fast as does the strength ratio. When the stiffness ratio is 1.0, the strength ratio is about 0.5. The stiffness of a healing fracture proceeds toward normal more quickly than does the strength. Thus, it should not be assumed from clinical assessments of fracture site rigidity that the fracture has returned to normal strength and can thus withstand unprotected loading.

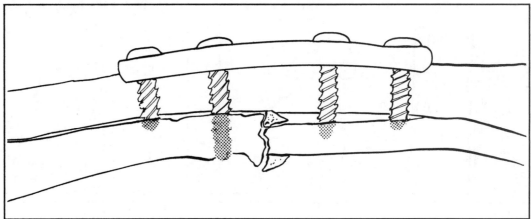

Slide V,59

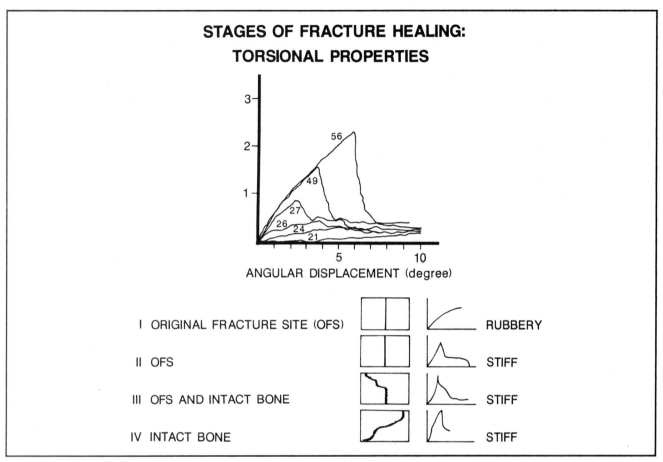

Slide V,60

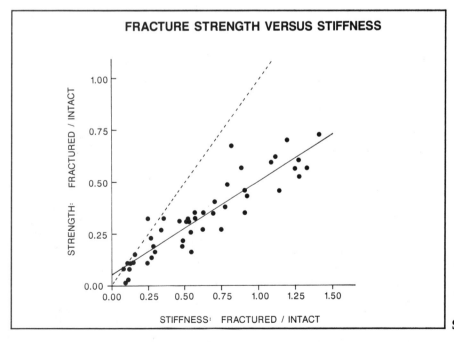

Slide V,61

Flexor Tendon Healing:
Strength and Excursion Properties

Three factors contribute to the formation of adhesions: tendon suture; digital sheath injury; and immobilization. In the laboratory, an *in vivo* model analogous to the clinical situation has been developed using a canine forepaw that produces "adhesion-free" healing. The flexor tendons are lacerated and repaired. Early intermittent passive motion is used to augment the repair process.

The strength of the tendons has been evaluated by tensile testing, as illustrated in Slide V,62. The early intermittent passive-motion group (Group III) achieves the greatest strength at the repair site, as compared to the immobilization group (Group I) and the delayed mobilization group (Group II). Gliding functions of repaired tendons are also affected by immobilization. Slide V,63, shows the effect of immobilization (Group I), delayed mobilization (Group II) and intermittent passive mobilization (Group III) on the repaired flexor tendon of the dog forepaw within its sheath. Both six weeks and twelve weeks after repair, the gliding properties of the mobilized tendon (Group III) are superior.

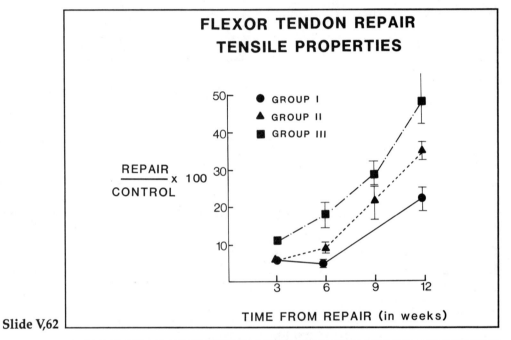

Slide V,62

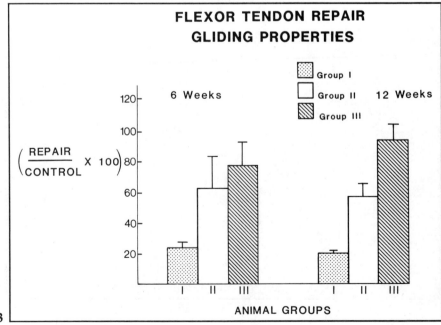

Slide V,63

The nature of the repair site in the area of early increased strength and the late effects of possible altered vascularization to the tendon because of early motion are as yet unknown.

Medial Collateral Ligament Healing

The medial collateral ligaments (MCLs) of rabbits were experimentally severed but not repaired. Studies of the healing process were performed up to 40 weeks post-operation. Representative biomechanical data obtained from tensile testing of the MCL-bone structure are shown in Slide V,64. As compared with the controls, the failure load of the MCL-bone structure is significantly lower for all healing ligaments. A gradual increase in the load at failure is noted with respect to time of healing. However, an apparent plateau in strength is reached at 14 weeks (60% of control), with no further increase evident.

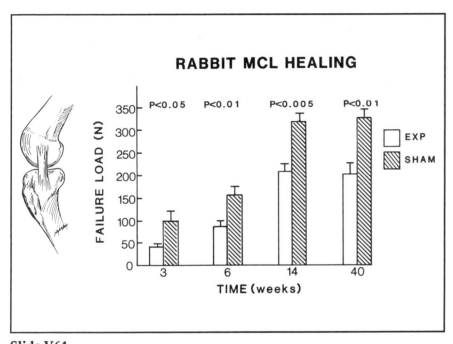

Slide V,64

Harrington Rod: Viscoelastic Stress Relaxation

In Slides V,24 and V,25, it was shown that a vertebral motion segment exhibits a pronounced viscoelastic stress-relaxation response when stretched or compressed. The left side of Slide V,65 illustrates the placement of a Harrington rod onto the spine of a person with scoliosis. A given amount of stretch is imposed onto the spine by the attachment hooks. The middle of the slide illustrates the mechanical viscoelastic spring and dashpot analog for the spine/Harrington rod configuration. Such a mechanical system will exhibit a stress-relaxation behavior. The initial force required to stretch the spine will gradually decrease in time due to the intrinsic viscoelastic behavior of the spine.

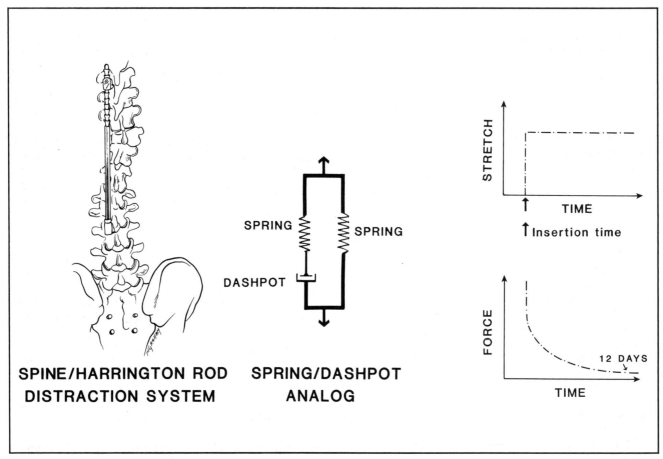

SPINE/HARRINGTON ROD
DISTRACTION SYSTEM

SPRING/DASHPOT
ANALOG

Slide V,65

Selected Bibliography

General

Bigland B, Lippold OJC: The relation between force, velocity, and integrated activity in human muscles. J Physiol 1954; 123:214.

Cochran GUB: A Primer of Orthopaedic Biomechanics. New York, Churchill-Livingstone, 1982.

Frankel VH, Burstein AH: Orthopaedic Biomechanics. Philadelphia, Lea and Febiger, 1970, chap 2,3.

McLish RD, Charnley J: Abduction forces in the one-legged stance. J Biomechanics 1970; 3:191.

Radin EL, Simon SR, Rose RM: Practical Biomechanics for the Orthopaedic Surgeon. New York, John Wiley and Sons, 1978.

Bone

Carter RS, Hayes WC: Bone compressive strength: The influence of density and strain rate. Science 1976; 194:1174-1175.

Frost HM: A determinant of bone architecture: The minimum effective strain. Clin Ortho 1983; 175:286-292.

Hayes WC, Carter DR: Biomechanics of bone, in Simmons D, Kunin A (eds): Skeletal Research. New York, Academic Pres, 1979.

Maquet PG, Van de Berg AJ, Simoret JC: Femorotibial weight-bearing areas. Experimental determination. J Bone Joint Surg 1975; 57A: 766.

Morris JM: Biomechanics of the spine. Arch Surg 1973; 107:418.

White AA, III, Panjabi JM: Clinical Biomechanics of the Spine. Philadelphia, JB Lippincott Company, 1978.

Joint

Akeson WH, Amiel D, Woo S L-Y: Immobility effects on synovial joints. The pathomechanics of joint contracture. Biorheology 1980; 17: 95-110.

Behrens JC, Walker PS, Shoji H: Variations in strength and structure of cancellous bone at the knee. J Biomechanics 1974; 7:201.

Frankel VH: Biomechanics of the knee. Orthop Clin North Am 1971; 2:175.

Goodfellow J, O'Connor J: The mechanics of the knee and problems in reconstructive surgery. J Bone Joint Surg 1978; 60:358.

Greenwald AS, Haynes DW: Weight-bearing areas in the human hip joint. J Bone Joint Surg 1972; 54B:157.

Kempson GE: Mechanical properties of articular cartilage, in Freeman MAR (ed): Adult Articular Cartilage. New York, Grune and Stratton, 1979, p 197.

Krause WR, Pope MH, Johnson R, et al: Mechanical changes in the knee after meniscectomy. J Bone Joint Surg 1976; 58A:599.

Lucas DB: Biomechanics of the shoulder joint. Arch Surg 1973; 107:425.

Mankin HJ: The reaction of articular cartilage to injury and osteoarthritis. N Eng J Med 1974; 291:1285.

Mankin H, Thrasher AZ: Water content and binding in normal and osteoarthritic human cartilage. J Bone Joint Surg 1975; 57A:76.

Mansour JM, Mow VC: On the natural lubrication of synovial joints: normal and degenerate. J Lubrication Tech 1977; 99:163.

Mansour JM, Mow VC: The permeability of articular cartilage under compressive strain and at high pressures. J Bone Joint Surg 1976; 58A:509.

Morris JM: Biomechanical aspects of the hip joint. Orthop Clin North Am 1971; 2:33.

Mow VC: Biphasic rheological properties of cartilage. Bull Hosp Joint Dis 1977; 38:121.

Radin EL, Paul IL: A consolidated concept of joint lubrication. J Bone Joint Surg 1972; 54A:607.

Radin EL: Biomechanics of the knee joint. Its implication in the design of replacements. Orthop Clin North Am 1973; 4:539.

Torzilli PA, Mow VC: On the fundamental fluid transport mechanisms through normal and pathological articular cartilage during function. II. The analysis, solution and conclusions. J Biomechanics 1976; 9:587.

Walker PS: Human Joints and Their Artificial Replacements. Springfield, IL, Charles C Thomas, 1977.

Walker PS, Erkman JJ: The role of the menisci in force transmission across the knee. Clin Orthop 1975; 109:184.

Walker PS, Hajek JV: The load-bearing areas in the knee joint. J Biomechanics 1972; 5:581.

Woo SL-Y, Akeson WH, Jemmott CF: Measurement of nonhomogeneous, directional mechanical properties of articular cartilage in tension. J Biomechanics 1976; 9:785.

Ligament

Akeson WH, Woo SL-Y, Amiel D, et al: Rapid Recovery from Contracture in Rabbit Hindlimb. Clin Orthopaedics and Rel Res 1977; 122:359-365.

Akeson WH, Woo SL-Y, Amiel D, et al: Biochemical and biomechanical changes in the periarticular connective tissue during contracture development in the immobilized rabbit knee. Conn Tiss Res 1974; 2(4):315-323.

Brantigan OC, Voshell AF: The mechanics of the ligaments and menisci of the knee joint. J Bone Joint Surg 1941; 23:44.

Hsieh H-H, Walker PS: Stabilizing mechanisms of the loaded and unloaded knee joint. J Bone Joint Surg 1976; 58A:87.

Hughston JC, Cross MJ, Andrews JR: Classification of lateral ligament instability of the knee. J Bone Joint Surg 1974; 56A:1539.

Hughston JC, Andrews JR, Cross MJ, et al: Classification of knee ligament instabilities. Part I: The medial compartment and cruciate ligaments. J Bone Joint Surg 1976; 58A:159.

Hughston JC, Andrews JR, Cross MJ, et al: Classification of knee ligament instabilities. Part II: The lateral compartment. J Bone Joint Surg 1976; 58A:173.

Noyes FR, DeLucas JL, Torvik PJ: Biomechanics of anterior cruciate ligament failure: An analysis of strain-rate sensitivity and mechanisms of failure in primates. J Bone Joint Surg 1974; 56A:236.

Noyes FR, Torvik PJ, Hyde MS, et al: Biomechanics of ligament failure. J Bone Joint Surg 1974; 56A:1406.

Noyes FR, Groud ES: The strength of the anterior cruciate ligament in humans and Rhesus monkeys. J Bone Joint Surg 1976; 58A:1074.

Trent PS, Walker PS, Wolf B: Ligament length patterns, strengths and rotational axes of the knee joint. Clin Orthop 1976; 117:263.

Woo SL-Y, Gomez MA, Akeson WH: The time and history dependent viscoelastic properties of canine medial collateral ligaments. J of Biomechanical Engineering 1981; 103(4): 298.

Woo SL-Y, Akeson WH, Amiel D, et al: The connective tissue response to immobility: A correlative study of the biomechanical and biochemical measurements of the normal and immobilized rabbit knee. Arthritis and Rheumatism 1975; 18(3):257-264.

Tendon

Brand PW: Biomechanics of tendon transfer. Orthop Clin North Am 1974; 5:205.

Crisp JDC: Properties of tendon and skin, in Fung YC, Perrone N, Anliker M (eds): Biomechanics, Its Foundations and Objectives. Englewood Cliffs, NJ, Prentice-Hall, 1972.

Gelberman RH, Manske PR, Akeson WH, et al: Flexor tendon repair. J Orth Res 1986; 4:119-128.

Woo SL-Y, Ritter MA, Amiel D, et al: The biomechanical and biochemical properties of swine tendons—long term effects of exercise on the digital extensors. Conn Tiss Res 1980; 7:177-183.

Woo SL-Y, Gelberman RH, Cobb NG, et al: The importance of controlled passive mobilization on flexor tendon healing. A biomechanical study. ACTA Ortho Scan 1981; 52:615-622.

Chapter VI

Biomaterials

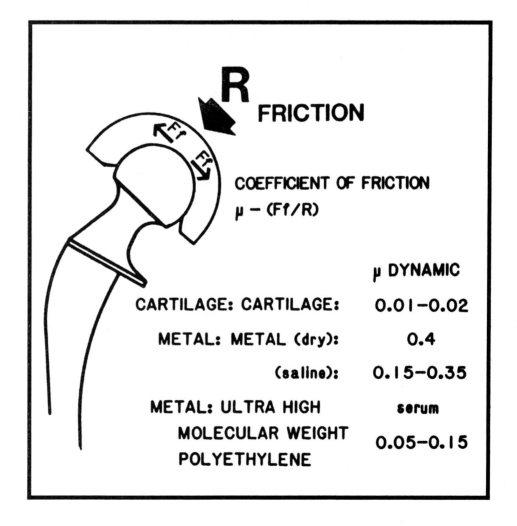

R FRICTION

COEFFICIENT OF FRICTION

$\mu - (Ff/R)$

	μ DYNAMIC
CARTILAGE: CARTILAGE:	0.01–0.02
METAL: METAL (dry):	0.4
(saline):	0.15–0.35
METAL: ULTRA HIGH MOLECULAR WEIGHT POLYETHYLENE	serum 0.05–0.15

The study of biomaterials centers on the relationship between physical structure and function in natural tissues and man-made biomaterials. This chapter discusses basic principles of material behavior, including deformation, fracture, wear, and corrosion, along with other degradation mechanisms of polymers, metals, ceramics and composites. Also discussed are biological responses to implanted man-made materials including a universal fibrous reaction, and osteolysis. The role of implant materials in inflammation and infection is also discussed.

Ultrastructure of Biomaterials

The physical properties of biomaterials depend on the nature of the chemical bonds between their atoms. The ultrastructure of biomaterials is illustrated in Slide VI,1. In metals, atoms form associations of closely packed positive ions with an associated "cloud" of electrons. Polymers are made up of long chains of carbon, nitrogen and other similar atoms held together by covalent bonds. Polymer chains are stabilized by weak associations between hydrogen and oxygen, called van der Walls' forces or by hydrogen bonds and occasional intermolecular bonds of other types. Ceramics consist of three-dimensional arrays of positively charged metal ions and negatively charged nonmetal ions, such as oxygen. These networks may be highly organized and crystalline, or disorganized and amorphous, or "glassy." Composites are usually formed by mechanical association of different materials with interdigitation of the materials and, in some cases, interface hydrogen bonds. This range of ultrastructures permits selection of diverse materials for medical uses.

Stress-Strain Behavior of a Material

Slide VI,2 illustrates the stress-strain behavior of a material. In the linear phase, stress is proportional to strain. In the plastic phase, stress is no longer proportional to strain. The stresses during which the material no longer behaves in a linear manner, (with stress no longer proportional to strain) is called the proportional limit (σp).

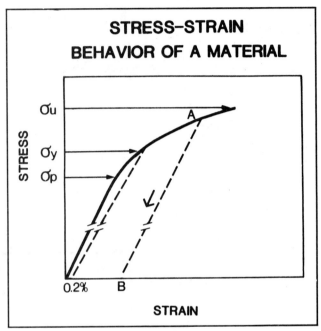

Slide VI,2

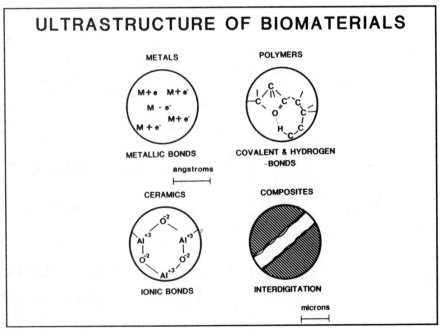

Slide VI,1

Since it is difficult to measure accurately the proportional limit, as a convention, a line offset at a strain of 0.2% and parallel to the initial linear region of the stress-strain curve is constructed; the corresponding stress at which the offset line and the original curve intersect is defined as the yield stress (σy). If the stress is removed from the material (point A), the elastic deformation (linear portion of the curve) is recovered, but the plastic deformation is not; the material is permanently deformed (point B).

Materials such as polymethyl methacrylate and most ceramics fracture very near the proportional limit. These materials are called "brittle" in that they do not undergo any significant permanent deformation prior to fracture. Many other materials, including cortical bone and most metal alloys, continue to deform beyond the proportional limit. These materials are "ductile."

Two important properties that can be measured by a stress-strain curve are toughness and ductility (Slide VI,3). Toughness is defined as the *energy supplied* to a material to cause it to fracture and is measured by the total *area* under the stress-strain curve. Ductility is the *total strain* (elastic and plastic) that a material can withstand prior to fracture.

Each class of materials has a characteristic stress-strain curve, as illustrated in Slide VI,4. Ceramics at room temperature are strong, brittle materials. They possess high moduli, very little plastic deformability at room temperature, and high compressive strength. Metals are strong, ductile, tough materials. They have relatively high moduli combined with significant plastic deformability and high energies of failure. Polymers have low moduli with ductility. Adding a strong, stiff material to a polymer results in a composite with increased stiffness and strength but with decreased ductility.

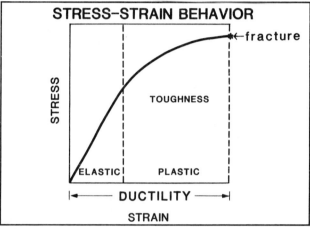

Slide VI,3

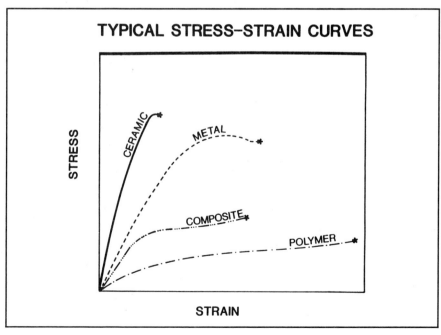

Slide VI,4

Fatigue

The graphic representation of fatigue behavior is shown in Slide VI,5. If a specimen is repeatedly loaded, even though the applied stress is below the yield strength of the material, the material can fail. This is called "fatigue failure." For many materials, if the stress is low enough fatigue failure will not occur. The maximum stress below which fatigue failure will never occur regardless of the number of cycles is known as the "endurance limit" of the material. Fatigue behavior is strongly influenced by environmental conditions. A corrosive environment, such as body fluid, can greatly reduce the number of cycles to failure and the endurance limit.

Fatigue failure will occur in any device in which the combination of local peak stress and number of cycles at that stress are excessive. Examples of fatigue failure are breakage of cerclage wires, prostheses and fixation hardware. In biologic tissues, bony stress fractures and certain tendon ruptures are additional examples.

Creep

The application of a load (stress) produces immediate elastic deformation (strain). In certain materials, continued application of the constant load produces *increasing* deformity with time. This time-dependent behavior, referred to as "creep," can be divided into three stages (Slide VI, 6). The primary stage is characterized by a high but decreasing rate of strain. A constant strain rate then follows in the secondary stage of creep. During the tertiary stage, a rapidly increasing rate of strain immediately precedes failure. Increasing load (stress) and increasing temperature will increase the amount of creep.

Many biomaterials, particularly polymers and most organic tissues, reflect elastic and viscous properties. The initial strain is produced by elastic deformation of the primary bonds of the macromolecules. Creep then reflects the viscous behavior produced by the "flow" of molecules resulting from the failure of secondary intermolecular bonds. Creep, sometimes called "cold flow," is partially recoverable after load release, but produces permanent deformation that may affect mechanical function, as in total joint replacements with polymeric components.

Stress Relaxation

When a material is deformed within the elastic limit, internal stresses are immediately produced. In materials such as metals and ceramics, constant deformation produces constant internal stress. In other materials, particularly polymers and biologic tissues, the *internal stresses decrease with time*, as shown in Slide VI,7. This relaxation of stress reflects the viscous nature of these materials in much the same way as creep behavior. Stress relaxation increases with increasing initial strain and increasing temperature. Stress relaxation in bone may contribute to early loosening of bone plates and spinal instrumentation.

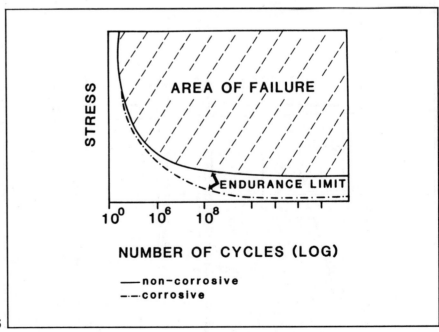

Slide VI,5

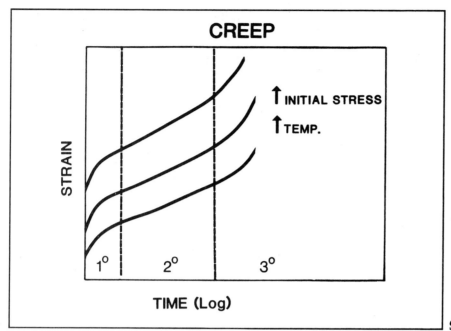

Slide VI,6

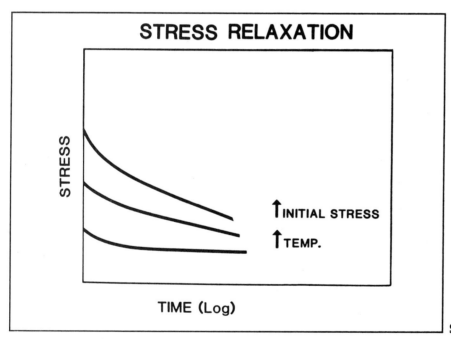

Slide VI,7

Bone Tissue Mechanical Properties

In most clinical situations bone acts as an elastic material similar to metal; however, bone tissue is actually visco-elastic; its mechanical behavior is time-dependent. As seen in Slide VI,8, if bone is stretched at different rates of strain, it will display different stress-strain curves. A specimen tested at a higher strain rate will exhibit a higher elastic modulus, yield stress, and ultimate stress than one tested at a lower strain rate. Bone rapidly loaded, such as in a high-speed motor vehicle accident, will withstand greater loads than when loaded slowly, such as in a fall in the lift line at a ski slope. Unfortunately, the ductility will be less at high deformation rates, and if a fracture occurs comminution is frequent.

The mechanical properties of bone *tissue* whether from cortical bone or cancellous bone are the same. Cortical and cancellous bone *structures* exhibit different properties for two reasons: l) the amount of bone tissue per unit volume (density) is different in the two structures; and 2) the arrangement and location of the bone tissue architecture is different. In general, the ultimate strength of bone structures (cortical or cancellous) is proportional to the density squared (ρ^2), while the elastic modulus is proportional to bone density cubed (ρ^3), as shown in Slide VI,9. Knowledge of such relationships will allow determination of bone's physical properties from the clinical assessments of bone density.

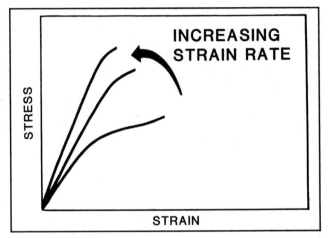

Slide VI,8

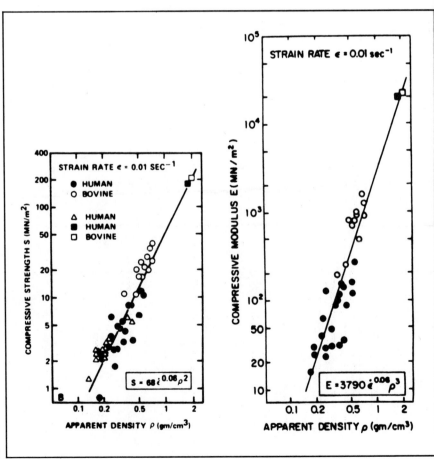

Slide VI,9

Strain-Related Potentials In Bone

Slide VI,10 indicates schematically the result of a four-point bending experiment on a rat femur. When the load is applied and immediately released, an electrical potential is produced. Upon loading, the concave side of the cortex, which is in compression, is negative with respect to the convex or tensile side of the cortex. Upon release, the potential decays rapidly to zero, reverses in sign and then again decays more slowly back to zero. If on the other hand, the load is applied and maintained, the electrical potential rises as before, but decays to a value of perhaps 10% to 30% of its peak value. This potential, called an "off-set potential," will be maintained more or less constantly for long periods, so long as the deformation of the bone is maintained. When the load is released, there is again a reversal of sign followed by a decay back to a zero potential difference.

These strain-related or "piezoelectric" potentials are produced by the organic components of bone and are not dependent upon cell viability. Live bone also displays fixed polarizations or "biopotentials" with increased negativity associated with regions of high cellular activity such as occurs in the epiphyseal plate or healing fracture. Collectively, these electrical effects are believed to be important in natural mediation of bone growth, repair and remodeling.

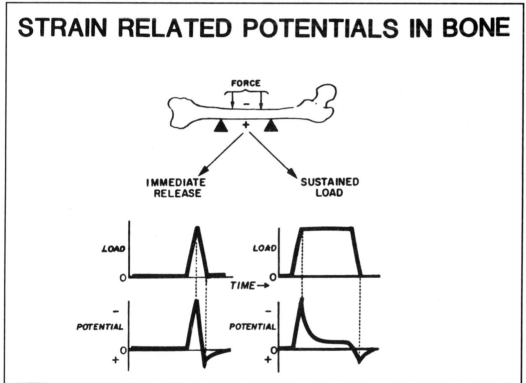

Slide VI,10

Mechanical Properties of Tendon/Ligament

The mechanical properties of tendon/ligament are discussed in Chapter 5, Biomechanics.

Problems in accurately measuring cross-sectional area and changes in length make it difficult to develop reliable stress-strain curves for soft tissues like tendon and ligament. Tendons and ligaments are usually tested as complete structures, with the resultant curves called load-deformation curves rather than stress-strain curves. The shape of the resulting load-deformation curve includes an initial "toe" region, followed by a linear region in which load is proportional to deformation, followed finally by the onset of failure. In the "toe" region, the stiffness is increasing, presumably due to the recruitment of more and more initially kinked fibers that straighten and begin to accept their share of the load. In the linear region, all fibers are straight and stretching in an elastic manner. Eventually, individual fibers begin to fail; failure progresses until all fibers have failed, at which time the entire ligament/tendon structure separates. As is bone, liga-ments and tendons are viscoelastic and their load-deformation curves are time-dependent. If an anterior cruciate is loaded rapidly, a stiff or brittle ligament tears in midsubstance. If loaded slowly, the ligament pulls away from its bony attachments.

Metal Alloy Systems

The chemical compositions of four common implant metals are depicted in the pie charts on Slide VI,11. Like all steels, stainless steels are predominately composed of iron. They achieve their corrosion resistance from substantial additions of chromium; whereas the addition of carbon and nickel add to their strength. The most common type of stainless steel used for implants is 316L but others are available. For example, a cast type specified A296 in the American Society for Testing and Materials Specification is used to make complex shapes where high strength is not necessary, such as the joint surface in total knee prostheses.

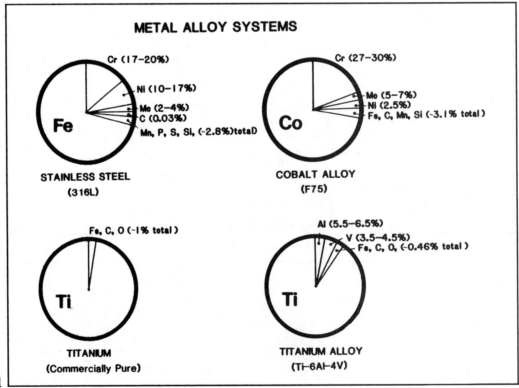

Slide VI,11

Cobalt alloys have a variety of trade names. Alloys predominately composed of cobalt are generally used in either the cast or wrought form, with significant additions of tungsten in the wrought form to provide ductility. A high nickel-content cobalt alloy, MP35N, also has multiple trade names. MP35N exceeds the cast and wrought cobalt alloys in yield stress, ultimate stress and fatigue strength. However, its high nickel content (35%) has raised questions concerning biological response, as nickel is biologically very active. Titanium is used both in its commercially pure form and alloyed principally with aluminum and vanadium. The mechanical properties of the alloy are far superior to those of the pure form of titanium.

Elastic Moduli of Metal Alloys

As shown in Slide VI,12, the elastic moduli of metal alloys used for implants are an order of magnitude higher than that for cortical bone. Among the implant metals, only titanium and titanium alloy differ, having moduli approximately half that of the stainless steels and cobalt alloys.

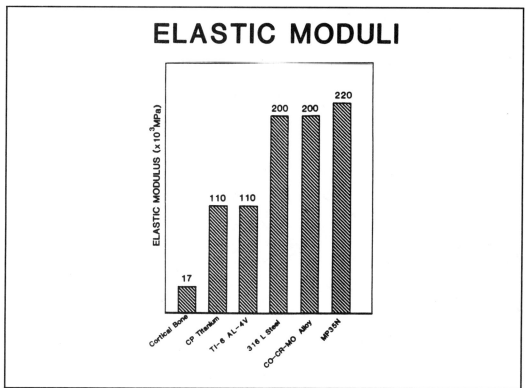

Slide VI,12

Strength Properties of Metal Alloys

The ultimate stress and the endurance limit of metal alloys used for implants vary considerably. Endurance limit is an important consideration in implant design, since implants are subjected to cyclic (fatigue) loading. Fatigue failure is related to endurance limits. As endurance limits are easier to measure, they are more commonly used to test new implants. (See Slide VI,13.)

Cold Working of Metal Alloys

A method used to improve the strength properties of metal alloys is "cold working." The metallurgical ultrastructure produced by mechanically deforming the material beyond its yield stress will exhibit superior yield and ultimate stresses with higher endurance limits. Unfortunately, because a large component of the deformation is permanent (or "plastic"), the remaining ductility of the material will be reduced. Slide VI,14 illustrates these properties.

Processing of Cobalt Alloys

The mechanical properties of a material are linked to its ultrastructure. Recently, two methods of processing cobalt alloy have been introduced into the orthopaedic marketplace. Hot isostatic pressing (HIP) is a process by which cobalt alloy powder is consolidated at high temperatures under constant pressure to create a fine-grained material. Forging is a process by which a blank of cobalt alloy is heated and pressed into a die of near final shape by the application of a large, single force. Both processes result in mechanical properties far superior to those of cast cobalt alloy.

Corrosion

Corrosion, the gradual degradation of materials by chemical attack, is identified most closely with the reactions between fully reduced metals and electrolyte solutions. As depicted in Slide VI,15, these reactions can be grouped into three general areas:

Corrosion—reactions that produce dissolved metal ions in concentrations greater than 10^{-6} molar.

Passivation—reactions that produce surface coatings, usually metal oxides of low solubility producing equilibrium solutions of metal ions in concentrations less than 10^{-6} molar.

Immunity—reactions that prevent the release of free ions in concentrations greater than 10^{-6} molar by the formation of stable surface compounds.

Corrosion is a very important phenomenon which provides the stimulus for many different biological responses.

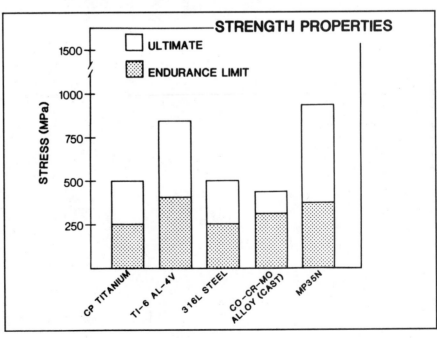

Slide VI,13

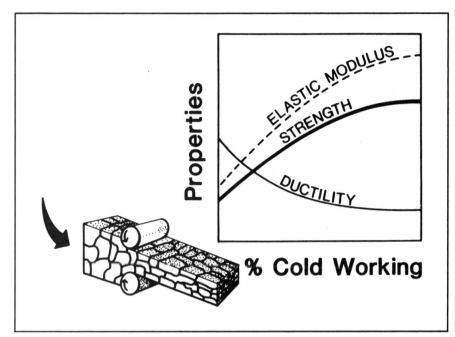

Slide VI,14

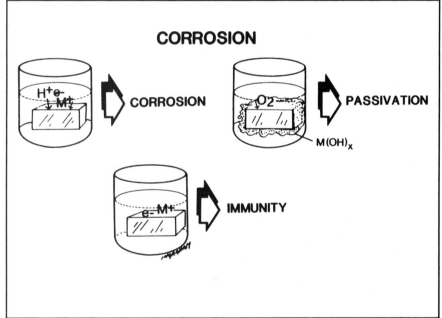

Slide VI,15

The Role of Hydrogen Ion (H+) and Oxygen (O₂) in Corrosion

Whether corrosion, passivation, or immunity occurs in a single part of a homogeneous metallic implant depends upon the pH and the oxygen tension present at the implant site. These conditions may be summarized in a pH-potential or Pourbaix diagram. Slide VI,16 illustrates the Pourbaix diagram for chromium, the oxygen-containing compounds of which are responsible for the passivation of both stainless steels and cobalt base alloys. Generally, tissue conditions are such that chromium-bearing alloys with preformed oxide layers are inactive *in vivo*. Some tissue locations, and occasionally transient conditions, such as the acid-pH shift associated with infection, may damage the chromium oxide layer and produce corrosion. Thus, a particular biomaterial may be well suited for one variety of implant application, but not for another. There is no such thing as a completely "biocompatible" material.

Types Of Corrosion

While all corrosion is dependent upon chemical reaction with or without oxidation/reduction, we can distinguish between several types of processes, as shown in Slides VI,17 and VI,18:

Uniform attack This process takes place under "corrosion" conditions on the Pourbaix diagram. Metal ions are released and either hydrogen(H+) or oxygen(O₂) free radicals serve as electron acceptors. A bathing solution with significant ionic conductivity such as that afforded by typical physiologic solutions is required.

Galvanic attack When two different metals are placed in contact in an electrolyte, preferential attack may occur on one member of the "couple." Differences in composition, amount of impurities or degree of cold working produce a higher degree of ionic release from one metal, termed the "base" or "anodic" member of the couple. Some of the electrons liberated flow to the other member, rendering it more "noble" or cathodic, thus protecting it from corrosive attack. In general, mixed metals in implants should be avoided. Of all the implant alloys in use, stainless steels are most likely to become anodic when in contact with other metals and thus to corrode preferentially.

Stress Corrosion Even passivated materials may suffer from general attack. The imposition of high tensile stresses may rupture the passive surface layers as well as rendering the underlying metal more chemically active. If conditions favor passivation, the cracks "heal" by reformation of the oxide layer. However, continued high cyclic stresses or the presence of organic molecules may interfere with formation of a new oxide layer (repassivation), and continued local attack can occur, leading to stress concentration and possible failure in load-bearing implants.

Intergranular attack If the impurities occur in aggregations between uniform volumes of alloy called "grains," then the attack focuses on these areas. The result is formation of intergranular grain-boundary cracks.

Crevice corrosion Defects such as scratches, interledges or seams may result in a linear attack, resembling pitting in mechanistic origins.

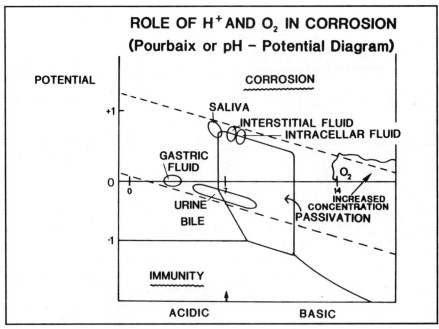

Slide VI,16

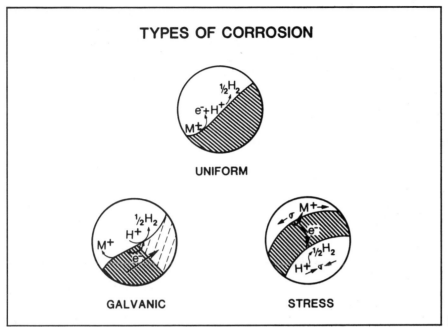

Slide VI,17

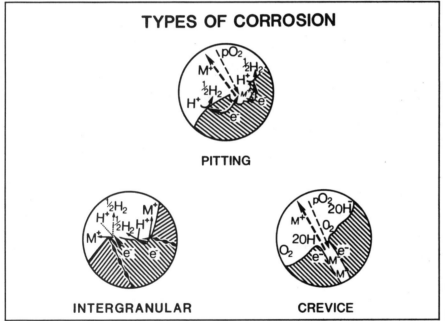

Slide VI,18

Chemical Degradation Of Polymers

Chemical attack modifies the degradation of polymers as well as metals, as illustrated in Slide VI,19. Absorption or loss of low molecular-weight molecules, such as water or lipids from a polymer will alter its mechanical properties. Reduction in the length of the covalent back bone of polymer molecules by oxidation, hydrolysis or chain-scission processes degrades mechanical behavior and increases solubility.

Slide VI,20 illustrates the relative sensitivity to chemical degradation of the four major synthetic biomaterials.

Metals, being fully reduced, are most subject to chemical attack. Polymers depend upon molecular weight for many of their properties and contain only partially oxidized atomic species. They are somewhat less susceptible than metals to chemical attack. Ceramics are essentially fully oxidized with high-energy ionic bonds and are relatively resistant to chemical degradation. The overall behavior of composites depends on both the properties of their individual components and upon the nature of their internal interfaces. They are therefore difficult to characterize. In the presence of adequate mechanical design, chemical degradation places the ultimate limit on the useful life *in vivo* of any biomaterial.

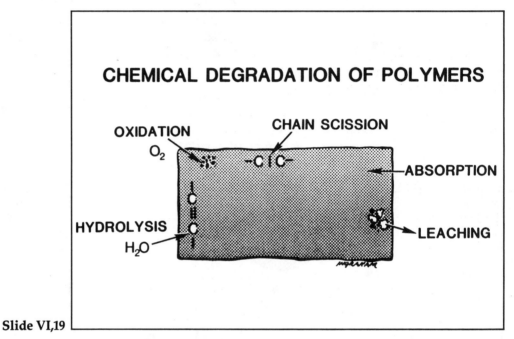

Slide VI,19

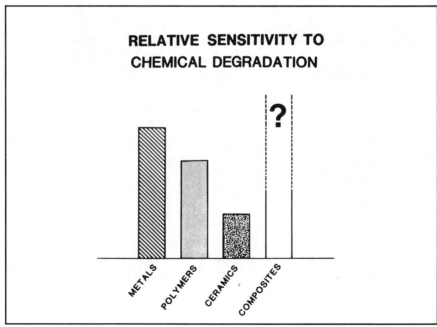

Slide VI,20

Friction

When two materials are in contact and in relative motion, a reaction or frictional force (Ff) exists that is proportional to the load across the interface, as illustrated in Slide VI,21. The ratio of these two forces is always less than one and is called the coefficient of friction (μ). When the relative motion first starts, the initial value is called "static fricion." As motion continues, the value of the coefficient decreases and is called "dynamic coefficient of friction." The purpose of lubrication is to reduce resistance to motion by providing minimum values of static and dynamic coefficients of friction for any pair of materials.

Lubrication Regimes

The nature of lubrication and, to a degree, its efficiency depend upon the lubricant, the separation of the two surfaces, and their relative velocity. In general, the more viscous the lubricant and the greater the separation of surfaces at a given relative velocity, the lower is the value of the dynamic coefficient of friction. In hydrodynamic lubrication (Slide VI,22), the surfaces are fully separated by the lubricant (h). In elastohydrodynamic lubrication, the elasticity of the bearing surfaces allows adaptation to surface irregularities without producing fatigue damage or plastic deformation. In mixed lubrication, the film is even thinner and surface damage may occur. Surface damage may be obviated by boundary lubrication in which surface binding of very "slippery"

films on smooth surfaces permits easy motion with little stress-concentration effect. If one or the other surfaces is porous, then the elastohydrodynamic regime is aided by fluid expression forming a pressurized lubricating mechanism called "weeping lubrication." Articular cartilage normally displays a combination of elastohydrodynamic, weeping, and boundary lubrication, while artificial joints display elastohydrodynamic and boundary lubrication.

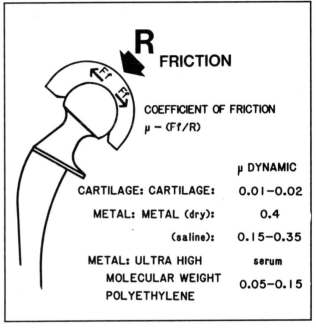

Slide VI,21

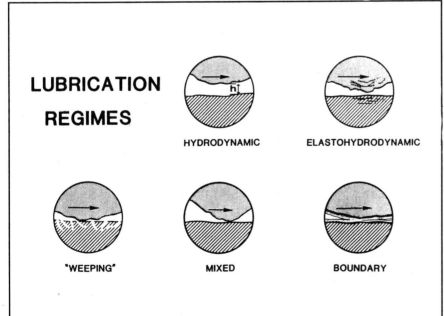

Slide VI,22

Wear Mechanisms

Lubrication acts to reduce frictional resistance and to separate surfaces so as to reduce local stress concentrations. Even in the face of low coefficients of friction, local surface interactions can produce local mechanical damage and loss of material. This process is called "wear." There are five important mechanisms of wear (Slide VI,23):

Adhesion Local binding of bumps or asperities subsequently can cause small pieces of the weaker material to be torn loose.

Abrasion ("plowing") If sufficiently large asperities (4 to 8 micrometers) exist on the stronger, harder side, they can plow through the softer material, producing needles and curls of loose debris, as a cutting tool produces on a lathe.

Transfer In some cases, a film of the softer surface may be transferred to the harder surface, changing the nature of the interface. Such transfer films are unstable.

Fatigue Local surface roughness on the hard side may not cause abrasion, but may produce sufficient subsurface stress concentrations in the softer material to produce fatigue failure. Such a surface has a characteristic microscopic net of cracks resembling a dried mud flat.

Third Body Trapping of wear debris within the moving interfaces or the introduction of foreign particles, such as bone or PMMA fragments, produces local stress concentrations that result in a combination of abrasive and fatigue wear.

Relative Wear Rates

Slide VI,24 illustrates that after an initial, high wear rate or wearing-in period, the volume of wear debris is proportional to the force across the interface and the total distance traveled. The proportional factor (Archard's constant) is dependent on the material, the lubricant, and the wear mechanism. In general, dissimilar material pairs show the lowest rates of debris production. Ceramic-polymer combinations produce the least amount of wear.

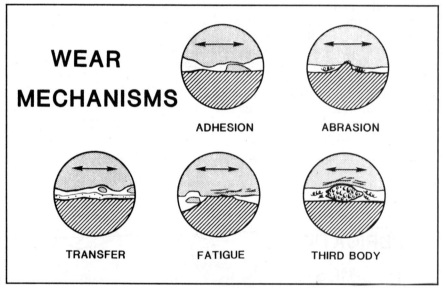

Slide VI,23

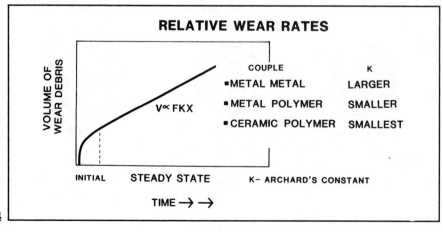

Slide VI,24

Properties Of Polymers

Slide VI,25 illustrates polymers commonly used in medicine. Several polymers have found important application in orthopaedics. Self-curing polymethyl methylmethacrylate (PMMA) is used as a grouting agent for joint replacement prostheses because of its ability to be formed *in vivo* prior to setting. Its modulus of elasticity is favorable for distributing strain to surrounding bone. However, PMMA strength is marginal for orthopaedic application and requires judicious use.

Ultra high-molecular weight polyethylene (UHMWPE) has found value as a bearing surface for joint replacement prostheses because of its relatively low dynamic coefficient of friction when articulated against metal. UHMWPE has relatively low strength and limited wear resistance, which pose potential problems.

The solution to certain clinical problems requires materials capable of withstanding large elastic deformation and able to absorb energy. Despite its low strength and poor wear behavior, silicone rubbers have found use as "spacers" to replace small load-bearing joints. Polyethylene terephthalate (Dacron) and polytetrafluoroethylene (teflon) are being used in fiber and woven forms for constructing artifical ligaments. The load-deformation behavior of the woven prostheses is beginning to approach the behavior of natural ligaments and tendons. However, strength remains an important issue.

In vivo fractures of polyethylene components for total joint replacement have been documented in the orthopaedic literature. Slide VI,26 shows an acetabular component that had been implanted for 76 months in a 79kg, 65-year-old man. At the revision operation, the component was found to be cracked at the base of the superior groove. Note that while polyethylene is a ductile material, the fracture in this instance has a brittle appearance. Microscopic examination of the fracture showed evidence of a fatigue mechanism.

PROPERTIES OF POLYMERS			
	ULTIMATE STRENGTH (MPa)	MODULUS OF ELASTICITY (MPa)	COMMENT
➡ POLYMETHYL METHACRYLATE (PMMA)	40	2000	GROUTING MATERIAL: SETTING IN VIVO
➡ ULTRAHIGH MOLECULAR WEIGHT POLYETHYLENE (UHMWPE)	40	1000	LOW COEFFICIENT OF FRICTION
➡ SILICONE RUBBER	5	---	ELASTOMER ABSORBS ENERGY
➡ POLYTETRAFLUOROETHYLENE (TEFLON)		500	---
➡ POLYPROPYLENE	35	---	---

Slide VI,25

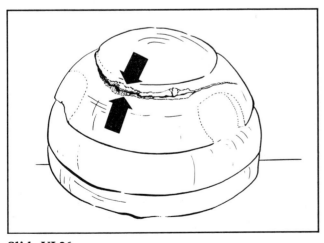

Slide VI,26

Practical Aspects Of PMMA (Bone Cement)

The properties of PMMA cements change dramatically during mixing and insertion into the surgical site, as illustrated in Slide VI,27. Immediately after mixing, at the initial doughy stage when it is "tacky," PMMA has relatively low viscosity, permitting intrusion into cancellous bone and anchoring holes. However, early insertion exposes the patient to elevated amounts of monomer release, producing the possibility of local cellular necrosis and systemic hypotension. Viscosity rises rapidly with time, so this intrusion capability is quickly lost. PMMA is not very "sticky" at any time. It supports implants rather than attaching them to bone. Even freshly mixed PMMA does not adhere well to itself or to old cement. The addition of irrigation fluid or blood further decreases this limited cohesion, as does time.

As the final stage of polymerization (setting) is reached, PMMA liberates significant amounts of heat. Large masses of cement reach higher surface temperatures than do small masses. Cellular necrosis and tissue damage at the cement-bone interface can occur from the heat given off during setting.

Ceramics And Carbons

Ceramics, particularly aluminum oxide, were initially commended as materials for the fabrication of implants on the basis of chemical inertness. Their relatively low tensile strength, high modulus, and brittleness have limited their value for the fabrication of orthopaedic devices. Recently, aluminum oxide has been found of value for the fabrication of articulating components of hip replacement prostheses because of its high resistance to wear and its low coefficient of friction when prepared with highly polished surfaces. Because of limitations in its mechanical properties, care must be taken in the fabrication and use of implants made from aluminum oxide. Some mechanical properties of ceramics and carbons are shown in Slide VI,28.

Carbon was also initially recommended as an implant material on the basis of its chemical inertness and perceived "biocompatibility." Initial studies suggested that tissue was more tolerant to the surface of carbon than to the surface of other biomaterials. Carbon is being investigated in two forms, graphitic and low-temperature isotropic (LTI). Graphitic carbon displays two-dimensional crystallinity and, therefore, anisotropic mechanical properties, whereas LTI carbon displays no ordered atomic structure.

Fibers of graphite display very high strength and modulus. Their strength and biocompatibility have led to their use in fabrication of prostheses for ligament and tendon repair. The brittle behavior of carbon fibers often leads to fragmentation with the subsequent formation of large amounts of particulate debris. Phagocytes engulf carbon fibers in much the same fashion as they do other materials and hence could initiate inflammatory and immunologic responses in the host. Attempts to limit this fragmentation by coating the carbon fibers with resorbable substances have not solved the problem.

LTI carbon has been investigated as a coating for metallic prostheses to render them more "biocompatible." Difficulties in the adherence of the carbon to metal substrates and questions about the local biological response to released particulate carbon prevent the widespread use of carbon implants at this time.

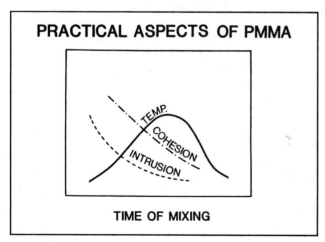

PRACTICAL ASPECTS OF PMMA

TEMP. COHESION INTRUSION

TIME OF MIXING

Slide VI,27

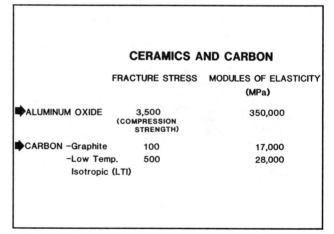

CERAMICS AND CARBON

	FRACTURE STRESS	MODULES OF ELASTICITY (MPa)
ALUMINUM OXIDE	3,500 (COMPRESSION STRENGTH)	350,000
CARBON –Graphite	100	17,000
–Low Temp. Isotropic (LTI)	500	28,000

Slide VI,28

Behavior Of Composites

Because of relatively low strength and modulus, polymers have limited use in the fabrication of load-bearing implants. As illustrated in Slide VI,29, this behavior can be improved by the addition of high-strength, high-modulus fibers, such as graphite fibers, to form a composite material. The reinforcement can be added as short, discontinuous fibers randomly oriented or as continuous fibers selectively oriented to provide properties that are dependent on direction. The choice of the fiber and its orientation provide opportunities to design materials with selected mechanical properties under different loading conditions, as seen in Slide VI,30. The effectiveness of the fiber reinforcement in increasing the strength and fatigue resistance is related to the bonding between the polymer matrix and the fiber. Coupling agents can be employed to obtain a chemical bond between the resin and fiber. Polymer bond composites are beginning to see use in highly stressed joint-prosthetic components and in low-stiffness (flexible) bone plates.

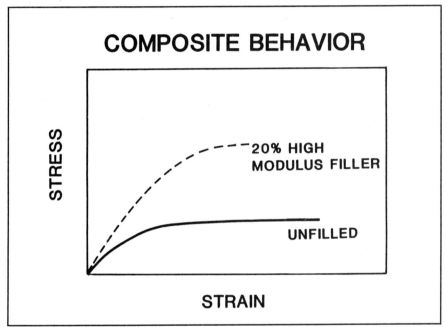

Slide VI,29

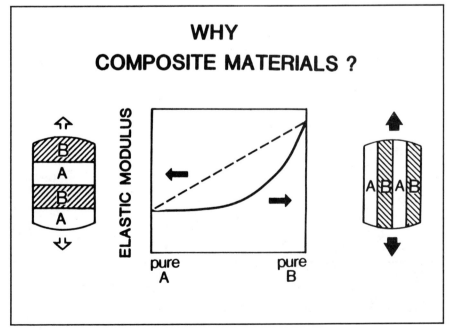

Slide VI,30

Biologic Response to Implants

Local Host Effects on Implants

The local host effects on implants can be exemplified by the subsequent loosening of the total knee implant shown in Slide VI,31 and the bone destruction about the femoral component of the hip implant in Slide VI,32. An understanding of what has occurred and how it might be avoided requires a knowledge of the biomechanical forces acting upon the prosthesis, knowledge of the material used in the prosthesis, and the patient's response to the biomaterial. Ideally, an implant should elicit little or no inflammatory response other than that caused by the implantation.

Local Host Response (Chronic, Normal)

The biologic reaction to implanted biomaterials includes local and systemic host responses, as shown in Slide VI,33. The cellular and tissue changes occurring in the vicinity of the biomaterial comprise acute and chronic phases. The cellular and extracellular events, constituting the transient acute phase, are consistent with the inflammation that occurs during the early stages of wound healing. Polymorphonuclear neutrophils, lymphocytes, and granulocytes can be found in the vicinity of the implant. Eventually macrophages and multinucleated foreign body giant cells can be found apposed to the surface of the biomaterial, perhaps adherent to the protein coat that forms on the surface immediately after implantation. Fibroblasts and the associated fibrous matrix, com-

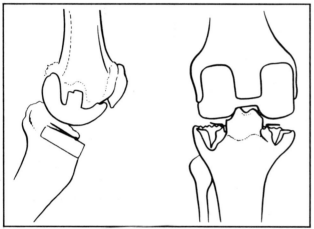

Slide VI,31

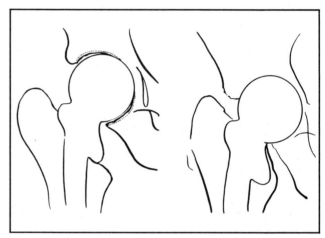

Slide VI,32

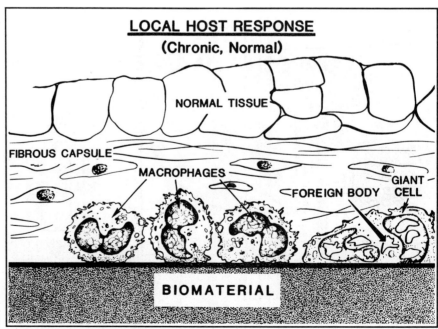

Slide VI,33

prising the "scar" is the result of the wound-repair process, encapsulating the implant. A continuing inflammatory response is elicited by the implant and consists of macrophages, giant cells and fibrous tissue. This chronic monocytic response is reminiscent of a foreign body granuloma and is maintained by the very presence of the implant. The thickness of this "fibrous capsule" and its cellularity are often used as a measure of the "reactivity" of the biomaterial. Local host response to infection about an implant can be found in Slide VI,34.

Features of the microenvironment created by the presence of an implant coupled with the selected adsorption of glycoproteins to the implant surface can predispose the implant site to bacterial infection. The presence of microorganisms at the implant interface can elicit an intense inflammatory response that destroys adjacent tissues. The presence of an implant can produce a "protected environment" for microorganisms. Host defense mechanisms and antimicrobial agents are less effective in the presence of the foreign material.

Clastic Response (Osteolytic Granuloma)

In the presence of biomaterials, cellular response can occasionally be so vehement as to destroy the bony tissue surrounding the implant. The clinical presentation of this response was shown in Slide VI,32 and is diagrammatically illustrated in Slide VI,35. Phagocytic cells responding to the presence of particulate matter from the biomaterials can directly attack surrounding bone or elaborate chemotactic or mitogenic factors that promote the invasion and destruction of the bone by other cells.

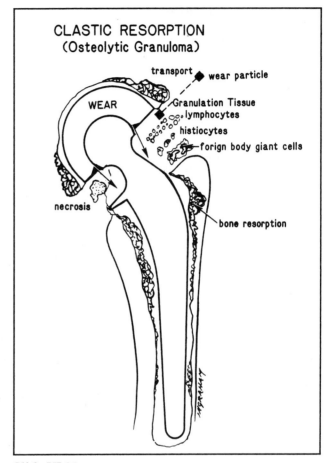

Slide VI,35

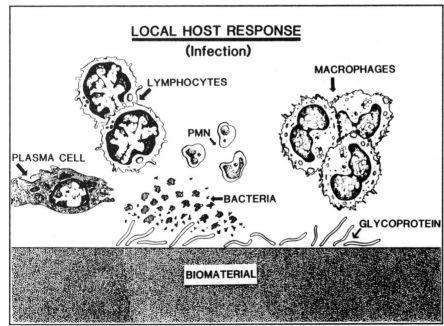

Slide VI,34

Neoplastic Transformation

The persistence of chronic inflammatory cells at the biomaterial surface can lead to the production of agents eliciting mutagenic and possibly carcinogenic changes locally and at distant sites, as suggested by Slide VI,36. Activated macrophages produce superoxide radicals that have been found to be mutagenic in fibroblasts.

The release of metal ions from the biomaterial can also lead to transformation of cells locally and at distant sites. Tumors such as malignant fibrous histiocytomas have been found in experimental animals and occasion-ally in humans with implants. A relationship between the tumor and the metal-releasing implants has been postulated but not proved.

Investigations using animals have demonstrated that selected cells found in the foreign-body response to biomaterials can undergo neoplastic transformation. It has been proposed that the pericyte (a small cell found adjacent to capillaries) can be a transforming cell, particularly in low-grade foreign body reactions in which low cellular activity levels prolong exposure for individual cells. The clinical relevance of these findings is unknown.

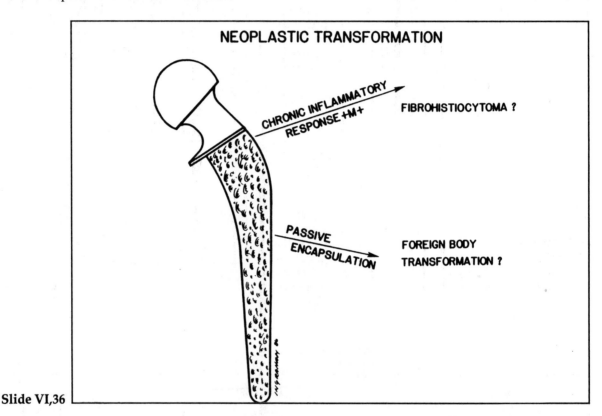

Slide VI,36

Systemic Response

Systemic responses are those responses produced distant to the implant site by blood-borne agents released by the biomaterial or by alteration in the host's molecules. This response is illustrated in Slide VI,37.

Complexes of protein, metal ions, and opsins can be presented by macrophages to T- and B- lymphocytes in the process of eliciting immunologic responses that can destroy tissue and produce a hypersensitivity reaction in the patient. In other cases, complement molecules such as C_3 can be cleaved as a result of interaction with the biomaterial surface. The activation of C_3 initiates an alternate pathway of the immunologic response that can also lead to tissue destruction. Additionally, metal ions released by the biomaterial can accumulate at sites distant from the implant. This accumulation can affect the normal metabolism and physiology of tissues and organs, as well as elicit tissue responses at distant sites usually associated with local host response.

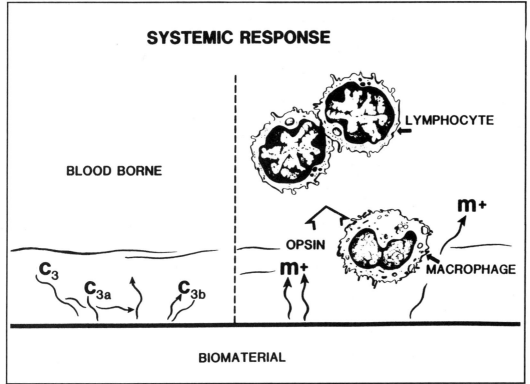

Slide VI,37

Systemic Effects

The body's rejection of foreign protein is a well-accepted fact, but the rejection of man-made implant materials has only recently attracted interest. Slide VI,38 illustrates loosening of a metalic hip nail in an individual who shows a positive skin test for sensitivity to one of the metals used in the nail. Slide IV,39 shows such a positive skin test. As more exotic materials and designs are introduced for human implantation, the clinician should be increasingly concerned about the possible systemic effects of these implants. The more surface area on the implant and the longer the implant remains within the body, the more opportunity exists for an adverse reaction.

Adaptive Remodeling

Osteoblasts and osteoclasts are influenced by the magnitude and state of strain imposed on them by loads applied to bone. See Slide VI,40. Stresses or strains within a given range seem to be required to maintain a steady-state remodeling of bone; i.e., formation rate equals resorption rate. Stresses below the minimum are often associated with "stress protection" leading to bone resorption. Stresses and strains exceeding upper limits can also produce resorption of bone as a result of "pressure necrosis."

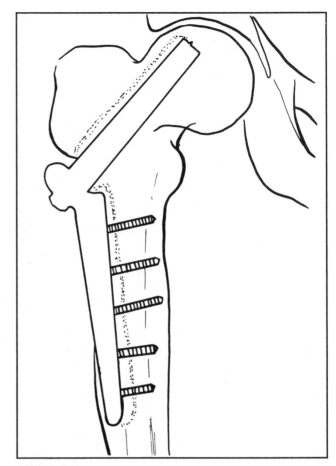

Slide VI,38

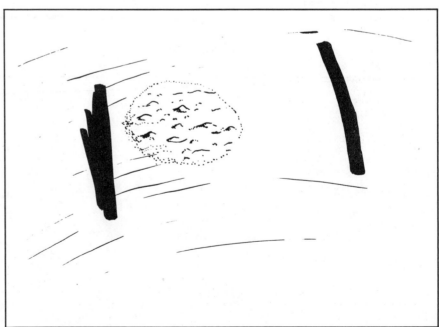

Slide VI,39

Observations of strain-related electrical potentials in bone, biopotentials, and electrical stimulation of osteogenesis combine to suggest a bioelectric phenomenon as the regulator of adaptive remodeling of bone. However, other investigations have shown that the strain imposed on the membranes of osteoblast-like cells in culture directly influences their activity, so other regulatory mechanisms are probably present in addition to electrical potentials.

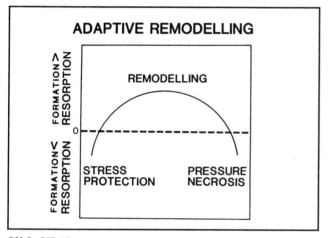

Slide VI,40

Adherence Of Bone To Biomaterials

The shear and tensile strength of a nonporous implant-bone interface is dependent on the attachment of bone to the implant. This attachment can result from mechanical interdigitation of bone with microscopic irregularities on the surface of an "inert" biomaterial or from the "chemical" bonding to bioactive substances.

Experiments with titanium implanted into bone have revealed that occasionally bone can grow close enough to the surface of the implant so that no fibrous layer seems to exist between the implant and the surrounding bone, as shown in Slide VI,41. This adaptation of bone to the surface of an implant without an interposed fibrous membrane is called osseointegration. This situation is *not* typical in current uncemented prosthetic implants.

"Direct bone bonding" has been evidenced on some biomaterials with calcium phosphate-rich surfaces. These "bioactive" materials include the minerals hydroxyapatite and whitlikite, and partially soluble "bioactive glasses" which form hydroxyapatite surface layers. Evidence suggests bioactive bone bonding produces a stronger interface with bone than does osseointegration (see the force displacement curve in Slide VI,41).

While there is considerable research interest in the use of osseointegration to supplant PMMA support in some applications, it is not in clinical use.

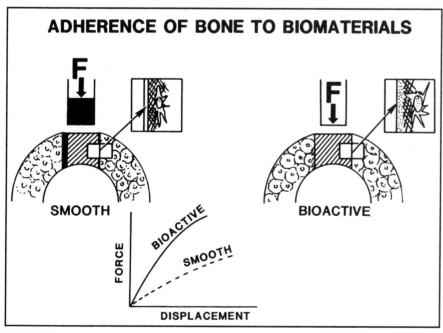

Slide VI,41

Bone Ingrowth Fixation

The bone ingrowth into a porous-surface coating on a joint replacement prosthesis leads to an interlocking bond that can serve to stabilize the implant. In order for the porous material to accommodate the cellular and extracellular elements of bone, the pore size must be above 100 micrometers.

The bone ingrowth process proceeds in two stages. The surgical trauma of implantation initially leads to the regeneration of bone throughout the pores of the coating. Then stress-induced remodeling leads to resorption of bone from certain regions of the implant and continued formation and remodeling of bone in other regions.

Porous coatings are most often produced by sintering techniques in which particles of the material are heat-fused to form a porous structure. The application of porous metal coatings to metallic stems can lead to reduced fatigue life because of changes in the microstructure produced by the high-temperature sintering of the coating or because the bonding of elements of the coating to the stem produces notches, which concentrate stress. Furthermore, the increased surface area provided by porous metals and the absence of a PMMA sheath around the metallic implant provide the host tissue with significantly more contact with the metal. The use of porous metals in young patients will allow many years for the accumulation of metal ions and an opportunity for their effects to appear.

Thus, despite considerable current interest in uncemented porous-coated total joint replacements, many issues of biological response remain unresolved.

Selected Bibliography

Stress and Strain

Bechtol CO, Ferguson AB, Laing FG: Metals and Engineering in Bone and Joint Surgery. Baltimore, The Williams and Wilkins Co, 1959, chap 6.

Cochran GUB: A Primer of Orthopaedic Biomechanics. New York, Churchill-Livingstone, 1982, chap 1.

Dumbleton JH, Black J: An Introduction to Orthopaedic Materials. Springfield, IL, CC Thomas, 1975, chap 2.

Frankel VH, Burstein AH: Orthopaedic Biomechanics. Philadelphia, Lea and Febiger, 1970, chap 2,3.

Levinson IJ: Mechanics of Materials, ed 2. Englewood Cliffs, NJ, Prentice-Hall Inc, 1970.

Williams DF, Roaf R: Implants in Surgery. London, WB Saunders Co LTD, 1973.

Properties of Materials

Cochran GUB: A Primer of Orthopaedic Biomechanics. New York, Churchill-Livingstone, 1982, chap 2.

Dumbleton JH, Black J: An Introduction to Orthopaedic Materials. Springfield, IL, CC Thomas, 1975, chap 3.

Hayden HW, Wulff J: The Structure and Properties of Materials. John Wiley Inc, New York, III, 1965, chap 1,4,7,8.

Nash WA: Strength of Materials. New York, McGraw-Hill, 1957.

Van Vlack, LH: Elements of Materials Science, ed 2. Reading, PA, Addison-Wesley, 1967, chap 4,6.

Viscoelasticity

Cochran GUB: A Primer of Orthopaedic Biomechanics. New York, Churchill-Livingstone, 1982, pp 91-96.

Coletti JM, Akeson WH, Woo SL-Y: A comparison of the physical behavior of normal articular cartilage and the arthroplasty surface. J Bone Joint Surg 1972; 54:147.

Dumbleton JH, Black J: An Introduction to Orthopaedic Materials. Springfield, IL, CC Thomas, 1975, chap 4.

Flugge V: Viscoelasticity. Waltham, Blaisdell Co, 1967, chap 1.

Frankel VH, Burstein AH: The viscoelastic properties of some biological materials. Ann NY and Sci 1968;146:158.

Frankel VH, Burstein AH: Orthopaedic Biomechanics. Philadelphia, Lea and Febiger, 1970.

Tissue

Ascenzi A, Bell GH: Bone as a Mechanical Engineering Problem, in Bourne GH (ed): The Biochemistry and Physiology of Bone. New York, Academic Press, I, 1972, chap 9.

Barbenel JH, Finlay JB: Stress-Strain-Time Relations for Soft Connective Tissues, in Kenedi RM (ed): Perspectives in Biomedical Engineering. Baltimore, University Park Press, 1973, p 165.

Bassett CAL: Biologic Significance of Piezoelectricity. Calcified Tissue Res 1968;1:252.

Black, J: Electric Stimulation: Its Role in Growth, Repair and Remodeling of the Musculoskeletal System. Praeger, 1986.

Dumbleton JH, Black J: An Introduction to Orthopaedic Materials. Springfield, IL, CC Thomas, 1975, chap 5.

Cochran GUB: A Primer of Orthopaedic Biomechanics. Churchill-Livingston, 1982, pp 113-127, chap 5.

Evans FG: Mechanical Properties of Bone. Springfield, IL, CC Thomas, 1973.

Freeman MAR (ed): Adult Articular Cartilage. New York, Grune and Stratton, 1973, chap 6.

Frost HM: Orthopaedic Biomechanics. Springfield, IL, CC Thomas, 1973.

Hastings GW, in Ducheyne P (ed): Natural and Living Biomaterials, CRC Press, 1984.

Yamada H, in Evans FG (ed): Strength of Biological Materials.

Wilkes GL, Brown, IA, Wildnauer RH: The biomechanical properties of skin. CRC Critical Reviews in Bioengineering, August 1973; p 453.

Metals

American Society for Testing and Materials, Annual Standards, 13.01, 1975.

Asher M, et al (eds): Orthopaedic Update I. Chicago, IL, American Academy of Orthopaedic Surgeons, 1984, chap 11.

Bechtol CO, Ferguson AB, Laing PG: Metals and Engineering in Bone and Joint Surgery. Baltimore, Williams and Wilkins, 1959.

Cochran GUB: A Primer of Orthopaedic Biomechanics. New York, Churchill-Livingstone, 1982, pp 96-105.

Dumbleton JH, Black J: An Introduction to Orthopaedic Materials. Springfield, IL, CC Thomas, 1975, pp 177-193, 192-194.

Williams DF, Roaf R: Implants in Surgery. London, WB Saunders Co, LTD, 1973, chap 2.

Corrosion

Cochran GUB: A Primer of Orthopaedic Biomechanics. New York, Churchill-Livingstone, 1982, pp 105-107.

Cohen J: Corrosion testing of orthopaedic impants, J Bone Joint Surg 1962; 44A:307.

Dumbleton JH, Black J: An Introduction to Orthopaedic Materials. Springfield, IL, CC Thomas, 1975, chap 7.

Fontana MG, Greene, ND: Corrosion Engineering. New York, McGraw-Hill, 1967, chap 4,5.

Sanlly JC: The Fundamentals of Corrosion. Pergamon Press, 1966, chap 2,4.

Friction, Wear and Lubrication

Cochran GUB: A Primer of Orthopaedic Biomechanics. New York, Churchill-Livingstone, 1982, pp 128-141.

Ducheyne P, Hastings GW (eds): Functional Behavior of Orthopaedic Biomaterials, II, CRP Press, 1984, chap 3.

Dumbleton JH: The Tribology of Natural and Artificial Joints. Elsevier, North Holland, 1981.

Dumbleton JH, Black J: An Introduction to Orthopaedic Materials. Springfield, IL, CC Thomas, 1975, chap 6.

Evarts CM (ed): Interposition and implant arthroplasty. Ortho Clin North Am 1973; 4.

Frankel VH, Nordin M (eds): Basic Biomechanics of the Skeletal System. Philadelphia, Lea & Febiger, 1980, chap 2.

Lubrication and wear in living and artificial human joints. Proc Inst Mech Eng 1966-1967;181:3J.

Rabinowicz E: The Friction and Wear of Materials. New York, John Wiley Inc, 1965.

Scales JT, Lowe SA: Choosing materials for bone and joint replacement. Engineering Med 1972; 1:52.

Williams DF, Roaf R: Implants in Surgery. London, WB Saunders Co, Ltd, 1973, pp 103-111, 407-417.

Wright V (ed): Lubrication and Wear in Joints. Philadelphia, JB Lippincott Co, 1980.

Polymers, Ceramics, and Composition

Asher, et al (eds): Orthopaedic Knowledge Update I. Chicago, IL, American Academy of Orthopaedic Surgeons, 1984, chap 12,13

Block B, Hastings GW: Plastics Materials in Surgery. ed 2, Springfield, IL, CC Thomas, 1972.

Boretos JW: Concise Guide to Biomedical Polymers. Springfield, IL, CC Thomas, 1972.

Charnley J: Acrylic Cement in Orthopaedic Surgery. Baltimore, Williams and Wilkins Co, 1970.

Cochran GUB: A Primer of Orthopaedic Biomechanics. New York, Churchill-Livingstone, 1982, pp 197-l13.

Dumbleton JH, Black J: An Introduction to Orthopaedic Materials, Springfield, IL, CC Thomas, 1975, pp 184-192, 194-197.

Hench LL, Splinter RJ, Allen WC, et al: Bonding mechanisms at the interface of ceramic prosthetic materials. J Biomed Mater Res 1971; 5:117.

Biocompatibility

Black J: Biological performance and materials, in Fundamentals of Biocompatibility. New York, Marcel Dekker, 1961.

Dumbleton JH, Black J: An Introduction to Orthopaedic Materials, Springfield, IL, CC Thomas, 1975, chap 9.

Laing PG: Compatibility of biomaterials. Orthop Clin North Am 1973; 4:249.

Walker PS, Bullough PG: The effects of friction and wear in artificial joints. Orthop Clin North Am 1973; 4: 275.

Williams DF (ed): Biocompatibility of Orthopaedic Implants. I, II, CRP Press, 1982.

Chapter VII

Non-skeletal Disorders

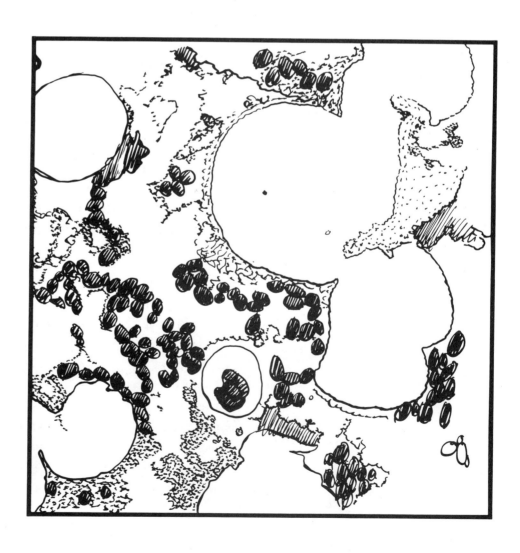

This chapter discusses conditions that affect organ systems other than the musculoskeletal system, but which are important to the orthopaedist in the management of patients. Discussions of musculoskeletal sepsis and immunobiology are also included, as both topics have important implications for the diagnosis and treatment of musculoskeletal disorders.

Thromboembolic Disease

Thromboembolism is frequently a lethal complication following musculoskeletal surgery. It is also the most common and dangerous of the complications occurring in patients sustaining skeletal trauma. The initiating mechanisms are obscure; clinical recognition can be elusive; and the recurrence rate is high. It has been estimated that thromboembolic disease results in 150,000 deaths annually in the United States. At least 750,000 are hospitalized annually with pulmonary embolism. The incidence of death from pulmonary embolism in England and Wales is shown in Slide VII,1. A geographic variation has been observed, with the problem occurring to a greater extent in the European countries and to a lesser extent in Africa, Asia, and South America.

Deep vein thrombosis has been found to occur in at least 50% of patients with fractures of the hip who undergo venography (Slide VII,2) or fibrinogen uptake, or both. In a study of patients undergoing total hip reconstruction, fatal pulmonary emboli occurred in 1.8% to 3.4% of patients. Approximately 50% of patients undergoing total hip replacement will develop deep vein thrombosis, as diagnosed by venography; 10% will develop

pulmonary embolism as diagnosed by lung scan; and approximately 2% of the patients will die from pulmonary emboli. A study involving 76 tibial fractures revealed a fatality rate from pulmonary embolism ranging from 0.5% to 1.3%.

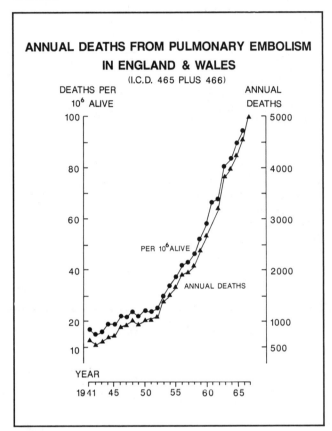

Slide VII,1

FREQUENCY OF THROMBOSIS
DIAGNOSED BY PHLEBOGRAPHY

AUTHORS PHLEBOGRAPHY		TRAUMA	FREQUECY OF THROMBOSIS (%)
●BORGSTROM ET AL	1965	HIP FRACTURES	56
●AHLBERG ET AL	1967	HIP FRACTURES	36
●FREEARK ET AL	1967	HIP FRACTURES	41
●JOHNSSON ET AL	1967	HIP FRACTURES	52
●HJELMSTEDT ET AL	1968	TIBIA FRACTURES	44
●MYHRE ET AL	1969	HIP FRACTURES	40
●HAMILTON ET AL	1970	HIP FRACTURES	49
●EVARTS ET AL	1971	HIP SURGERY	54
●FIELD ET AL	1971	HIP FRACTURES	62
●INWOOD ET AL	1973	HIP SURGERY	50

Slide VII,2

Coagulation

Clotting occurs by an enzymatic cascade of events, as depicted in Slide VII,3. There are three phases to blood coagulation: the first is the prothrombin-converting activity; the second is the conversion of prothrombin to thrombin by intrinsic and extrinsic pathways; and the third is the conversion of fibrinogen to fibrin. In this slide, note the central role of factor X and the influence of factor V and lipid upon the conversion of prothrombin to thrombin. The final phase in blood coagulation is a conversion of fibrinogen to fibrin, a loose clot initially followed by further activity in the presence of factor XII, which converts loose fibrin to tight fibrin.

Normal rate-limiting reactions occur as part of the blood-coagulation mechanism. These limiting reactions depend upon the appearance of specific inhibitors, the activation of fibrinolytic mechanisms and the consumption of coagulation factors. As shown in Slide VII,4, the fibrinolytic mechanism that is a normal component of the homeostatic mechanism involves the conversion of plasminogen to plasmin in the presence of tissue activators. Factor XIIa and thrombin produce plasmin with its action upon fibrin, factor V, factor VIII, and fibrinogen.

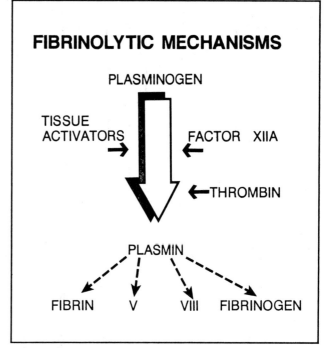

Slide VII,4

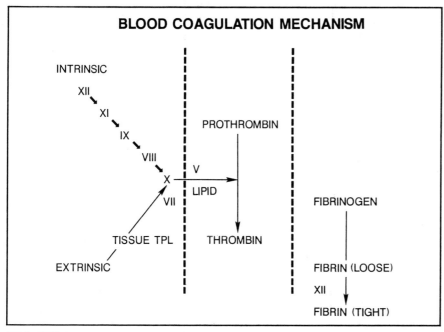

Slide VII,3

Pathogenesis of Thrombosis

There are postoperative changes that occur in patients who undergo musculoskeletal surgery. The same changes have been observed following skeletal trauma. The changes involve an increase in plasma procoagulant, an increase in fibrinogen levels, an increase in platelet reactivity, thrombocytosis, and on occasion, defective fibrinolysis. All of these changes "set the stage" for the development of a deep-vein thrombosis. There may be an increase in factors II, V and VII in the venous blood from the operative limb following total hip replacement. This increase may explain, in part, the high frequency of deep-vein thrombosis occurring following total hip surgery. A study done in 1968 revealed that 50% of the patients developed a thrombus during operation. This important discovery points to the need for prophylaxis.

If a clot begins during surgery or at the time of trauma, greater attention should be given to the administration of prophylactic agents before and during the operative procedure. It has also been observed that isolated deep-vein thrombosis occurs in the thigh more commonly after total hip replacement than after other forms of surgery. On other occasions, it has been clearly observed that clot formation begins in the popliteal veins and propagates proximally.

Recently, abnormalities of platelet adhesiveness and platelet survival times, as well as an alteration of fibrinolysis have been identified in the postoperative period. The available evidence suggests that the activation of a venous thrombosis may follow the formation of a small platelet nidus, as shown in Slide VII,5. The platelets accumulate behind the small valve cusp with progressive and successive layers of platelet and fibrin extending across the vessel causing a clot formation.

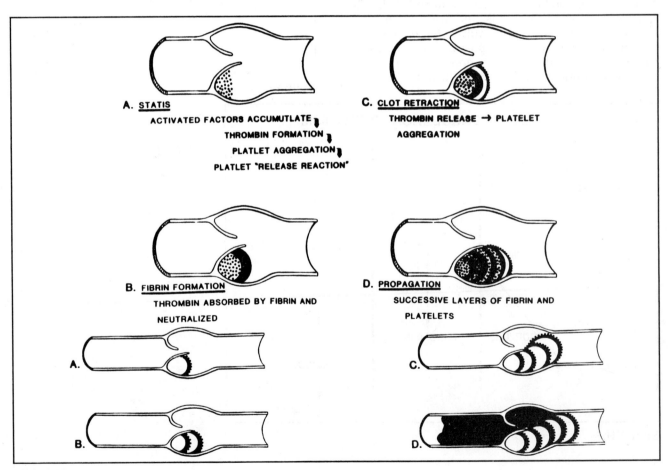

Slide VII,5

Currently, the thrombogenic factors recognized in the production of a clot are the platelets, the coagulation cascade, the fibrinolytic system, the vessel wall and the hemodynamics of blood flow through the venous system. The role of the platelet remains central in this process. As shown in Slide VII,6, factor X may be critical in initiating thrombin formation. Investigations have shown that the clinically significant thrombosis is composed of a large fibrin and red-cell coagulant and that an important reaction controlling thrombin formation may be the activation of factor X. The pathogenesis of venous thrombosis is summarized in Slide VII,7.

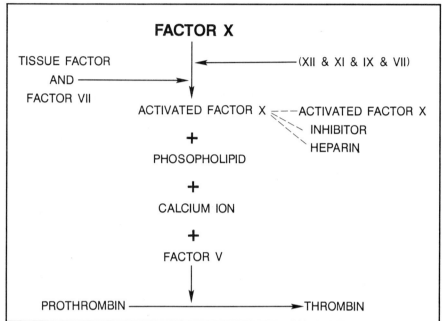

Slide VII,6

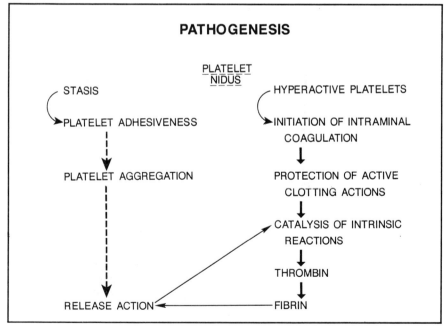

Slide VII,7

DIAGNOSTIC ACCURACY

VENOGRAPHY	97%
FIBRINOGEN UPTAKE	90%
ULTRASOUND	80%
IMPEDANCE	70%

Slide VII,8

Diagnostic Studies

There are many techniques utilized for detecting deep-vein thrombosis. These include clinical examination; venography; fibrinogen scan; tomography; and doppler ultrasonography. Slide VII,8 illustrates the relative accuracy of a number of methods of detecting venous thrombosis. Another technique for the detection of venous thrombosis in the lower extremity employs radioactive iodine-labeled fibrinogen. It is a noninvasive technique and reliable as a screening method. However, it is not accurate in the vicinity of a large wound, and is, therefore, impractical following major hip surgery. It does not detect thrombosis of the upper thigh, iliac or pelvic veins.

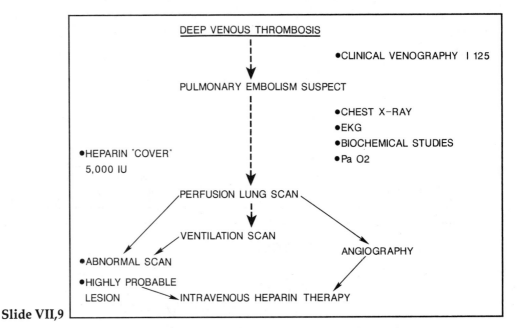

Slide VII,9

Slide VII,10

Other screening techniques, such as ultrasound impedance phlebography, have not been found to be as accurate as venography or I[125] labeled fibrinogen studies. Greater care must be taken to recognize the presence of pulmonary embolism. Slide VII,9 illustrates the diagnostic and therapeutic steps to be taken when pulmonary embolism is suspected.

Drug Actions

Drugs such as dextran, coumadin, heparin, and aspirin have been administered for the prevention of deep-vein thrombosis. The identification of the high-risk patient population is critical in regard to prophylaxis. High-risk patients include those with cardiovascular disease, pre-existing venous disease, or an underlying malignancy. Other high-risk factors include the presence of hematologic disorders, estrogenic therapy and obesity.

The anticoagulant coumadin has been shown in several studies to be an effective agent in preventing deep-venous thrombosis in the patient with a musculoskeletal disorder. The blood coagulation mechanism is affected by coumadin at the following levels: Factors IX, X, VII and the conversion of prothrombin to thrombin. (See the arrows on Slide VII,10.)

Heparin is an effective antithrombotic prophylaxis in certain patients. Currently, the use of low-dose heparin is not indicated for high-risk patients sustaining musculoskeletal injuries or undergoing major musculoskeletal procedures. The inhibitor to activated factor X (smaller arrow, Slide VII,10) is influenced even by trace amounts of heparin. Heparin increases the rate at which antithrombic factor VIII combines with factor X.

Dextran, aspirin, and dipyridamole have been used as platelet inhibitors. Aspirin *in vitro* reduces platelet adhesiveness to glass; reduces platelet aggregation; inhibits platelet aggregation induced by adenosine diphosphate, adenosin and thrombin; and inhibits prostaglandin production and prostacyclin synthesis. These latter two actions have a paradoxical effect on thrombosis. On the basis of available published data, there is no persuasive evidence that aspirin is completely effective in the prophylaxis of venous thromboembolism. It appears to be effective in the male in low doses, but has not been proved effective in premenopausal women or in high-risk patients.

Dextran has been used as a prophylactic agent. The available dextrans are glucose polymers of varying molecular weights. (Low molecular weight dextran = 40,000 average molecular weight; clinical dextran = 70,000 average molecular weight). The antithrombotic properties of dextran include a decrease in platelet adhesiveness, a change in fibrin clot structure, increased lability of thrombi, and blood flow improvement. Dextran can be effective in preventing fatal pulmonary emboli, but complications include congestive heart failure, renal failure, wound edema, hemodilution and allergic reactions. In the United States allergic reactions are rare. However, the effect of low molecular weight dextran and heparin are synergistic. If heparin must be administered, then only one-half to one-third the normal dosage should be given for the treatment of pulmonary emboli.

If thromboembolic disease is viewed as a pathologic process beginning with platelets and ending with thrombus dissolution, therapy beginning with physical measurements and ending with fibrinolytic agents is appropriate. Slide VII,11 illustrates the three classes of pharmaceuticals effective in preventing pulmonary embolism.

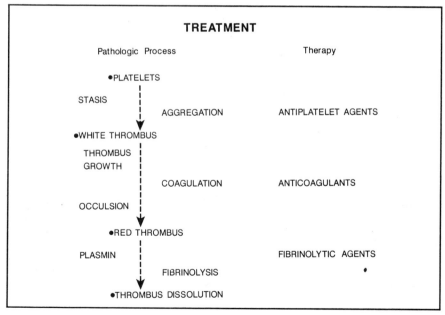

Slide VII,11

Shock

Shock is a clinical condition characterized by signs and symptoms that arise when the cardiac output is insufficient to perfuse vital organs and tissues. There are four categories of shock:hypovolemic; cardiogenic; vasogenic; and neurogenic. They result from the failure in the normal physiologic operation of one or more of the following interrelated mechanisms: 1) heart; 2) fluid or blood volume; 3) arteriolar resistance; and 4) capacity of the venous system. In shock secondary to hypovolemia, (VII,12B) the cardiac output falls and as a compensatory mechanism, the arteriolar sphincters contract, increasing the peripheral vascular resistance. At the same time, venous constriction is forcing more blood into the arterial side. In cardiogenic shock, (VII 12C) the heart is ineffective, leading to a loss of volume in the arterial system. To improve blood pressure, the peripheral vascular resistance is increased and because of the heart's failure as a pump, a tremendous amount of blood collects in the dilated venous system.

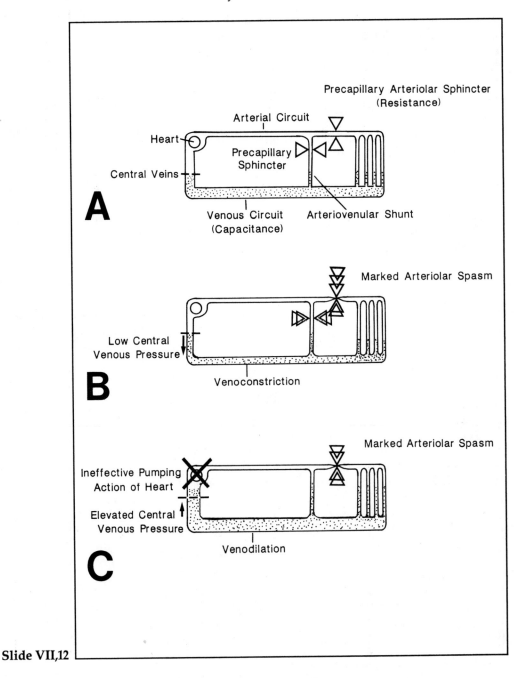

Slide VII,12

Shock developing from pulmonary embolism or pericardial tamponade produces its result by the same mechanism, i.e. a dilated nervous system and arteriolar constriction (Slide VII,13D.). Shock arising as a result of neurogenic or septic causes is characterized by venous and capillary dilatation with pooling of blood, loss of the sphincter tone in the arterioles, and open arterial venous shunts (VII, 13E).

Biochemical changes occurring in shock usually fall into three categories: 1) the pituitary-adrenal response to stress; 2) changes secondary to reduction in tissue perfusion; and 3) changes secondary to organ failure. The immediate effect of shock is adrenal sympathetic activity characterized by increased circulating epinephrine levels. This effect can be documented by the findings of eosinopenia, lymphocytopenia, and thrombocytopenia. At the same time, there is a striking negative nitrogen balance, retention of sodium and water, and increased excretion of potassium.

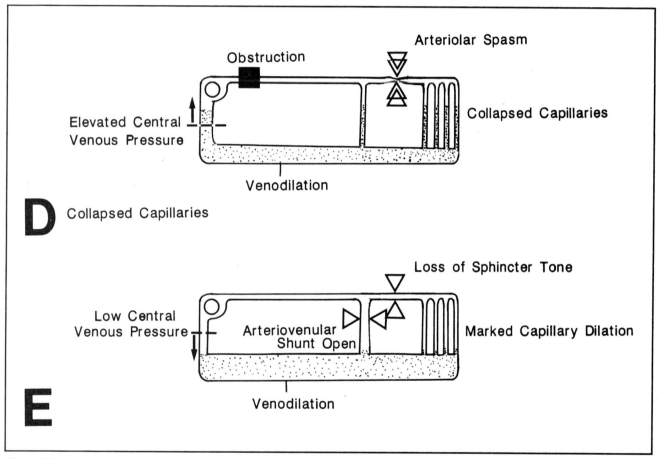

Slide VII,13

In the algorithm shown in Slide VII,14, the neurohumeral control of volume restitution is depicted. Hypovolemia stimulates baroreceptors in the right atrium, which relays impulses to the medullary nuclei and hypothalamus. The sympathetic nervous system then responds by causing vasoconstriction and stimulation of the adrenal glands, which releases cortisol and aldosterone, causing the kidney to retain fluids. Once initiated, these responses can be interrupted only by exogenous volume restoration in the form of intravenous fluids.

The changes secondary to the low-flow state have been shown to result in decreased oxygen delivery to vital organs and, consequently, in a shift from aerobic to anaerobic metabolism. The striking example of this shift is an increase in lactic acid production. There is a positive correlation between morbidity and the severity of the acidosis produced in shock. The major organ involved in shock is the kidney, as normally 25% of the cardiac output goes to the kidneys. The kidneys' response to hypovolemia is a release of renin by the juxtaglomerular apparatus. Renin, in turn, is converted to angiotensin, which stimulates aldosterone release from the adrenal glands. Finally, aldosterone increases tubular resorption of sodium and water in an attempt to restore fluid volume. Commonly, the renal response to shock includes a decreased glomerular filtration rate with retention of BUN and other waste products (Slide VII,15).

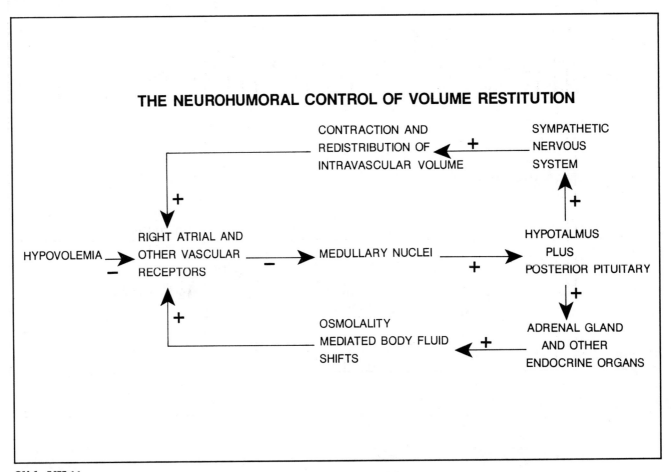

Slide VII,14

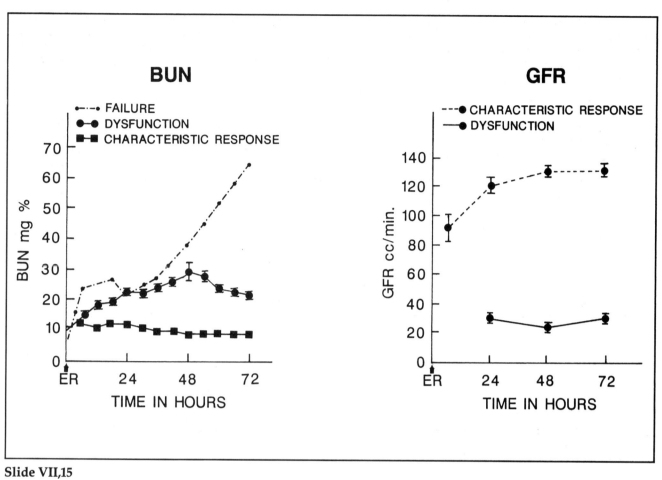

Slide VII,15

Acute respiratory failure after severe injury or shock may result in injury at the alveolocapillary membrane with leakage of proteinaceous fluid into the interstitium and alveolar spaces.

The liver is unusually susceptible to shock, with resultant changes of central necrosis and hepatocellular damage despite an increased blood flow in the hepatic artery compensating for the reduced flow in the portal vein caused by sphincter vasoconstriction. In the gastrointestinal tract, there is hemorrhage, edema and necrosis. An increase in the back diffusion of hydrogen ions through the gastric mucosa may lead to an acute ulcer attack and erosive gastritis.

In reversible hemorrhagic shock, the volume of extracellular fluid decreases. It shifts into the vascular tree and also, importantly, into the cells (Slide VII,16). As noted in Slide VII,17, survival is improved by using lactated Ringer's solution and blood replacement to restore extracellular fluid volume.

Additional evidence for these shifts of extracellular fluid has been found in experiments that studied the cellular membrane potential. As shown in Slide VII,18, the interstitial fluid potassium rises markedly and the cellular membrane potential is reduced. The changes appear to be reversible. The exact mechanism for producing these electrolytic changes and shifts in extracellular water is not understood.

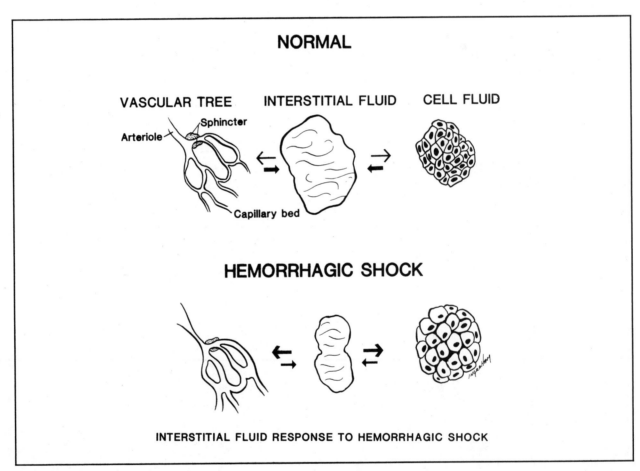

Slide VII,16

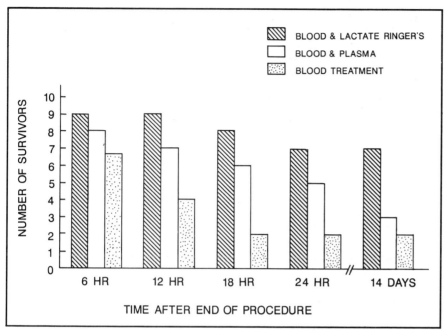

Slide VII,17

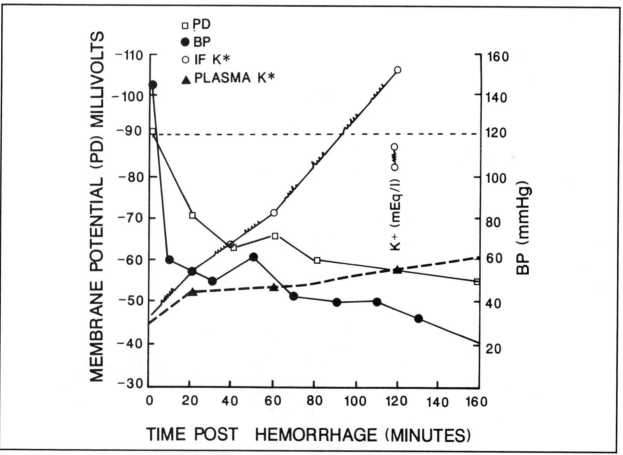

Slide VII,18

Adult Respiratory Distress Syndrome

The adult respiratory distress syndrome has the following hallmarks: l) hypoxemia relatively unresponsive to elevations of inspired oxygen; 2) decreased pulmonary compliance, i.e., a progressively increased airway pressure required to achieve adequate ventilation; and 3) chest radiographic changes from minimal to widespread areas of consolidation. Causes of hypoxemia include hypoventilation, diffusion defects, and ventilation/perfusion abnormalities such as shunting.

Slide VII,19 diagrams ventilation/perfusion abnormalities. Normal alveoli are shown at the top. In the middle right example, perfusion is adequate, but the alveoli are partially obstructed. In the middle left diagram, alveoli are aerated, but blood flow is diminished. Exchange of gases across the alveolocapillary membrane is impeded in both cases. The bottom left example shows normal aeration but no circulation, resulting in dead-space ventilation. Shunting is depicted on the bottom right: the circulation is normal, but the alveoli are not ventilated.

As shown in Slide VII,20, the possible causes of adult respiratory distress syndrome include pulmonary injury, infection, aspiration, fat embolism, microembolism, fluid overload, oxygen toxicity, microatelectasis, direct pulmonary injury, and cerebral injury. Recent data show that adult respiratory distress syndrome may be associated with fat embolism after isolated long-bone fracture, but the incidence is very low.

POSSIBLE CAUSES OF ARDS FOLLOWING INJURY

1. ISCHEMIC PULMONARY INJURY (?)
2. PULMONARY INFECTION
3. SYSTEMIC INFECTION (SEPSIS)
4. ASPIRATION
5. FAT EMBOLISM
6. MICROEMBOLISIM

7. FLUID OVERLOAD
8. OXYGEN TOXICITY
9. MICROATELECTASIS
10. DIRECT PULMONARY INJURY
11. CEREBRAL INJURY

Slide VII,20

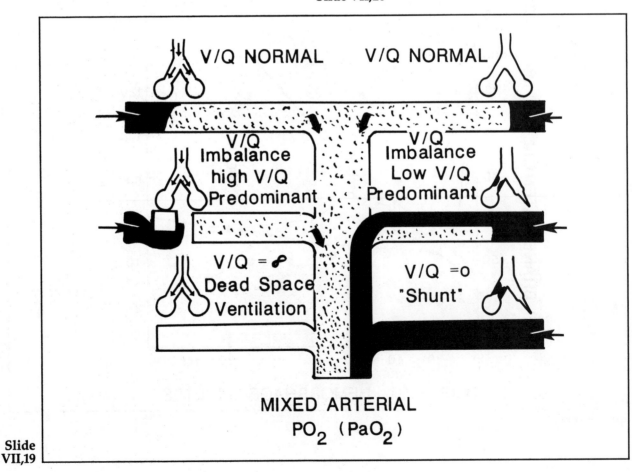

Slide VII,19

Fat Embolism Syndrome

The fat embolism syndrome is manifested clinically as an adult respiratory distress syndrome with progressive dyspnea and hypoxemia following skeletal trauma. Petechial hemorrhages are pathognomonic. The literature reports an incidence of 50% to 80% with a mortality of 10% to 20%.

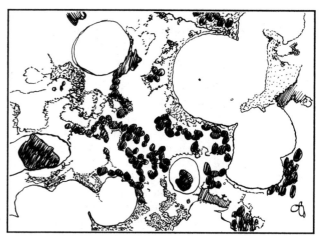

Slide VII,21

Three theories have been postulated to explain the pathogenesis of the fat embolism syndrome: 1) mechanical, as illustrated in VII,21, in which the fat released at the fracture site plugs the lung capillaries and breaks down into free fatty acids that are highly toxic to lung tissue; 2) metabolic, in which the post-traumatic hypovolemic state mobilizes fat from stores throughout the body and results in increased serum fats that break down into free fatty acids in the lung tissue; 3) centroneurogenic, in which a central nervous system abnormality caused by hypovolemia results in hypoxemia. Slide VII,22 summarizes these theories and the events occurring in the fat embolism syndrome.

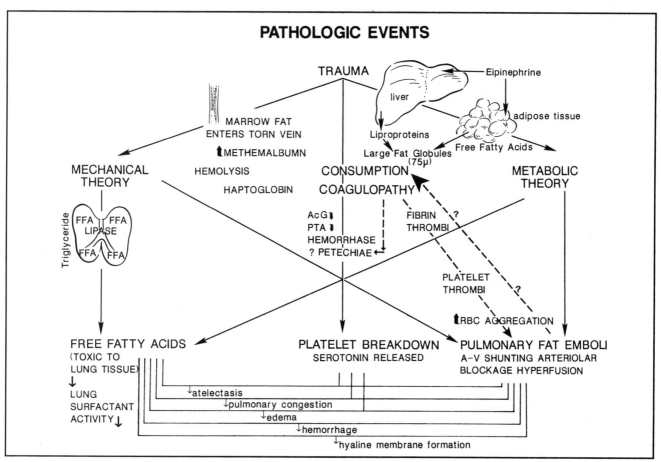

Slide VII,22

The pathophysiology of fat embolism is related to several factors. First, there appears to be a mechanical blockage of the pulmonary capillaries by fat, resulting in arteriovenous (AV) shunting and alveolar hypoperfusion producing hypoxia. Secondarily, inflammation occurs as neutral fats are broken down into free fatty acids by lipase contained in the lung. Finally, the platelets that are adherent and found among these fat globules break apart, releasing serotonin, which causes further vasoconstriction and bronchoconstriction, again leading to hypoxia. Free fatty acids are very toxic to lung cells, leading to disruption of the alveolocapillary membrane and lung surfactant (Slide VII,23), alveolar collapse, hemorrhage and edema—all resulting in a ventilation/perfusion deficit. The following factors may also contribute to the fat embolism syndrome: 1) the amount and type of embolic fat, such as arachidonic acid, which is so injurious to lung tissue that immediate death results; 2) shock; 3) severity of the injury; 4) host response to the injury; 5) abnormalities in platelet function; 6) abnormalities in the plasma clotting system.

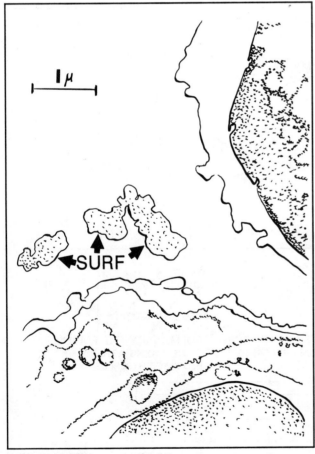

Slide VII,23

Hemoglobinopathies

The hemoglobinopathies are a group of disorders produced by an alteration in either the production rate or the structure of the globin portion of the hemoglobin molecule. The sickling disorders are the result of insoluble aggregates of hemoglobin S in the deoxygenated state. Red cells containing HbS_2 sickle when oxygen is removed.

The prevalence of sickle cell disease in the United States constitutes a major public health problem. Approximately 8% of American blacks have AS hemoglobin, while an estimated 0.2% have the homozygous SS state. Slide VII,24 shows the expected distribution of genotypes of various hemoglobin mating types. These distributions are based on mendelian inheritance modes.

Hemoglobin Chemistry

In the normal adult there are two B chains and two A chains and the hemoglobin tetramer is designated 2AB2A or HbA. The sickling phenomenon stems from a basic molecular defect, the substitution of valine for glutamic acid on the 6th position on each of the B-polypeptide chains. When hemoglobin S is deoxygenated, its solubility is markedly reduced and Hb aggregates or gels. This property makes Hb S vastly different from normal Hb A. Ultimately, the shape of the red cells is distorted into sickle or holly-leaf forms. Usually sickle cells will revert to normal shape upon reoxygenation. Repeated sickling induces sufficient membrane damage to certain susceptible cells so that the rigidity and sickle shape persist even after the cell has been reoxygenated and its hemoglobin is no longer aggregated.

The most common forms of sickle cell diseases are in descending order of severity and frequency: homozygous (sickle cell anemia); sickle cell hemoglobin C (Hb SC disease); and sickle cell-B+ thalassemia. Sickle cell disease causes a variety of clinical symptoms and signs that may be classified into five major groups: 1) chronic hemolytic anemia; 2) chronic organ damage; 3) anemic "crises"; 4) systemic manifestations; and 5) vaso-occlusive or painful "crises." As shown in Slide VII,25, bone infarcts are of major orthopaedic concern.

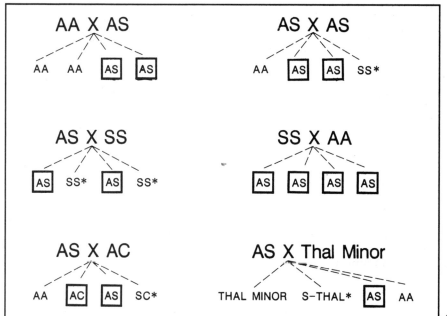

Slide VII,24

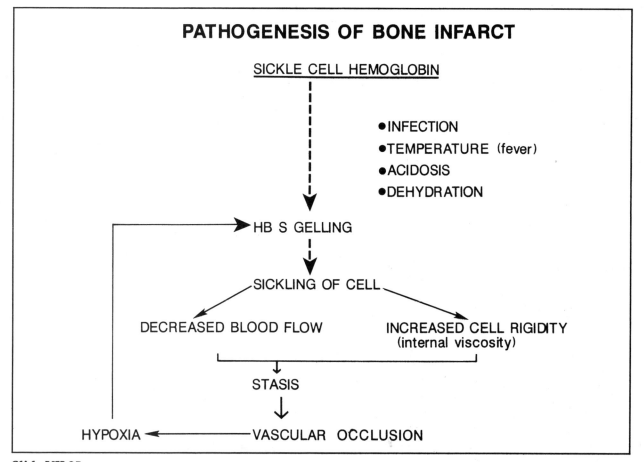

Slide VII,25

Pathophysiology of Musculoskeletal Sepsis

Osteomyelitis arises through one of four mechanisms: 1) hematogenous bacterial seeding of the medullary portion of a bone or joint; 2) open fractures or joint injuries following trauma; 3) seeding of the wound during elective surgical procedures; and 4) extension from an adjacent soft-tissue infection. (See Chapter 4, Pathology, for a discussion of osteomyelitis.)

Acute Hematogenous Osteomyelitis and Septic Arthritis

Blood-borne bacteria tend to lodge in the metaphyses of long bones. As discussed in the section on bone development in the anatomy chapter, the metaphyseal capillary loops at the physis play an important role in supplying blood to the physis. The ascending limb of the capillary loop is small (8 microns), the descending limb is large (15 to 60 microns). This sudden increase in diameter causes slow and turbulent blood flow, allowing bacteria to settle out of the mainstream and initiate infection.

Acute hematogenous osteomyelitis Two theories have evolved to explain the etiology of acute hematogenous osteomyelitis: mechanistic and physiological. The mechanist theory proposes that bacterial clumps occlude the nutrient artery, producing necrosis by infarction and secondary sepsis. The physiological theory suggests that a localized infection is initiated by the unique vascular supply to tubular bones and by an abnormality of phagocytic activity. Some theorists emphasize the importance of vascular occlusion and others have identified foci of traumatically induced thromboembolism in the initiation of acute hematogenous osteomyelitis. Abnormalities of the reticuloendothelial cells lining the capillary loops may facilitate initiation of the septic foci. Phagocytic cells, present only on the venous side of the capillary loop, exhibit weak phagocytic activity. These observations help to explain the propensity for infections in the metaphysis of tubular bones as compared to the rarity of infections in other organs with similar vascular loops and highly developed reticuloendothelial cells, such as the spleen and liver.

Once infection begins, bacterial toxins and the host's humoral and cellular responses combine to produce tissue necrosis. The resulting debris, exudate, and acidosis increase the local intraosseous pressure, further compromising blood flow and promoting more necrosis. The infectious process spreads through the paths of least resistance: the haversian system; Volkmann's canals; and the intramedullary space. Purulent material accumulates within the intramedullary canal and beneath the periosteum (via Volkmann's canals) to isolate all or a portion of the diaphysis from its vascular supply. That portion of the diaphysis deprived of its vascular supply becomes necrotic, forming a sequestrum. New periosteal and endosteal bone is formed to create an involucrum about the necrotic bone, the sequestrum (Slide IV,52-Pathology). Involucrum formation represents the host's attempt to isolate the infectious process. When the host's defense mechanisms fail to eradicate the microorganisms precipitating the infectious process, a Brodie abscess surrounded by a fibrous membrane and a wall of dense bone may develop. The infection may then become quiescent only to undergo recrudescence at some future date.

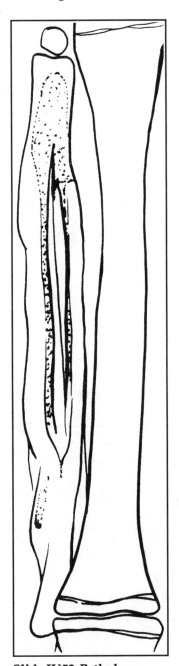

Slide IV,52-Pathology

If large sequestered pieces of cortical bone are isolated within the necrotic infected material contained by the involucrum, persistence of the infection can be anticipated. These sequestered pieces of cortical bone are avascular, precluding penetration through the vascular system by antimicrobial agents. The sequestrum provides a favorable environment for the microorganisms. Necrotic debris accumulates until sufficient pressure or cortical necrosis occurs to form a sinus tract. The sinus tract usually follows a sinuous course, emerging some distance from the central focus of the infectious process.

Acute hematogenous osteomyelitis is only rarely diagnosed in adults. The unique metaphyseal capillary loops disappear with obliteration of the physis at puberty. Typically, osteomyelitis occurs in patients whose host defense mechanisms have been compromised by disease or medications. Instrumentation may also introduce bacteria. Vertebral osteomyelitis may follow genitourinary tract instrumentation. In contrast to the *Staphylococcus aureus* usually seen in children, adult acute hematogenous vertebral osteomyelitis is usually caused by gram-negative bacteria.

In recent years, acute hematogenous osteomyelitis and septic arthritis have been encountered in adult patients who self-inoculate bacteria in the course of "shooting up" heroin. The individuals are usually men (male-female ratio: two to one). Infections in this group of patients occur most frequently in the sternoclavicular and sacroiliac joints and the lumbar and cervical vertebrae. *Pseudomonas aeruginosa* has been the most commonly isolated organism.

Septic Arthritis In acute septic arthritis in adults, loss of ground substance (glycosaminoglycan) appears to be the initial change in articular cartilage. Loss of glycosaminoglycans is usually not associated with visible alteration of articular cartilage until the collagen of the superficial tangential zone is destroyed (see discussion in Anatomy and Soft Tissue chapters). The latter was demonstrated to occur with use of the joint following loss of glycosaminoglycans. Synovial mediators, known as "catabolins," serve as local hormones to initiate chondrocyte catabolic destruction of matrix within articular cartilage. Once started, the degradative process does not require continued synovial stimulation. At this time the process can be interrupted only with the use of corticosteroids.

Post-traumatic Infections

Osteomyelitis as a sequel to traumatic injuries has become more prevalent because of the increasing magnitude and frequency of vehicular and industrial accidents. This group of patients often has fractures of the appendicular skeleton and extensive soft-tissue injury. The

alteration of the host's defense mechanisms permits bacterial colonization to produce subsequent infection at the fracture. In contrast to acute hematogenous osteomyelitis, in post-traumatic osteomyelitis, the diaphysis is affected more frequently than the metaphysis.

Whereas *Staphylococcus aureus* causes almost all cases of chronic hematogenous osteomyelitis, a more diffuse group of microorganisms has been isolated from patients with post-traumatic osteomyelitis. Contamination of traumatic wounds with soil or water, as well as microorganisms associated with nosocomial infections are responsible for this diffuse pattern of infection. *Staphylococcus aureus* remains the most frequently isolated organism (50% of patients). *Pseudomonas aeruginosa* has been isolated from 25% of patients. Almost half the patients with post-traumatic osteomyelitis have polymicrobic infections, usually composed of mixed gram-positive and gram-negative isolates. Anaerobic isolates account for 20% of the causal organisms. In general, the anaerobic isolates are recovered from mixed infections.

Postoperative Infections

Fortunately, most postoperative wound infections resolve with adherence to basic medical and surgical principles of debridement, drainage, and specific antimicrobial therapy. Chronic osteomyelitis is usually limited to those wounds containing an implant in or on osseous tissue. Chronic osteomyelitis in joint prosthetic surgery has been infrequent. Although infection following arthroplasty is not usually thought of as being osteomyelitic, the infection usually involves the osseous tissue located at the bone-cement interface of one or both components and, therefore, fulfills the definition of osteomyelitis.

The vulnerability of a total joint arthroplasty to postoperative infection may result from the acrylic cement used for fixation to osseous tissue. Monomeric methylmethacrylate, which leaches from curing polymethylmethacrylate, adversely affects leukocyte hemotaxis, phagocytosis, serum complement activity, and T-lymphocyte response. This alteration of the immune system may explain the prevalence of low-grade infections by microorganisms formerly considered to be "non-pathogenic," e.g., *Staphylococcus epidermidis*. Gram-negative bacillary organisms are distinctly uncommon.

Immunobiology

The immunologic response to foreign antigens is both humoral and cellular, as shown in Slide VII,26. The stimulation of specific lymphocytes, known as "B" and "T" cells, initiates the immune response. These cells arise from a basic bone-marrow stem cell, with T-cell development influenced by the thymus and B-cell development influenced by bursal cells (Slide VII,27). The T cells are primarily responsible for cellular immunity, while the B cells direct the humoral response by secreting antibodies.

CHARACTERISTICS OF THE IMMUNE SYSTEM		
	Humoral Immunity	**Cell-Mediated Immunity**
Response	Rapid	Delayed
Primary cell	"B" lymphocyte; plasma cell	"T" lymphocyte
Transfer of immunity	Immunoglobulins (antibody)	Lymphocyte (lymphokines)
Examples	*Anaphylaxis*	*Tuberculin type*
	Virus and toxin neutralization	*Delayed hypersensitivity*
		Allograft rejection

Slide VII,26

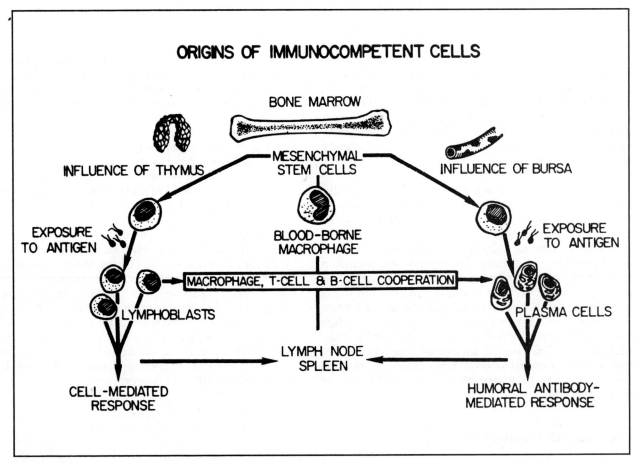

Slide VII,27

Antibodies are immunoglobulins produced by mature B cells and plasma cells (developed from B cells). The five classes of immunoglobulins are IgG, IgM, IgA, IgE, and IgD. All classes have the same basic structural subunits: two light and two heavy peptide chains linked by a disulfide bond (Slide VII,28). There are two groups of light chains (approximately 25,000 daltons):kappa and lambda. Almost two-thirds of the immunoglobulins of normal serum contain kappa chains, with the remaining containing light chains. There are five separate classes of heavy chains (50,000 to 75,000 daltons) that give rise to the five major divisions of immunoglobulins. Thus, while each immunoglobulin class corresponds to a specific heavy chain, all classes have either kappa or lambda light chains.

Within each immunoglobulin class, the amino acid sequence has terminal regions of variable heavy and light chains (VH and VL in Slide VII,28). The remaining part of the polypeptide chains is constant (CH and CL in Slide VII,28). The variable portion gives the immunoglobulin specificity to bind antigen, while the constant portion is not activated until antigen binding has taken place. The properties of the constant portions of each immunoglobulin vary.

Papain (Slide VII,28) cleaves immunoglobulins at the hinge regions to produce two identical antigen-binding fragments (Fab) and a third component (Fc). Pepsin digestion produces a single bivalent antigen-binding fragment (Fab)[2]. The Fc fragment fixes complement, crosses the placenta, and binds to macrophages.

The functions of each immunoglobulin are specific. IgG, the most abundant immunoglobulin in the extravascular space, fixes complement, binds to macrophages, crosses the placenta, and responds to most infectious and toxic agents. IgM, which is the first immunoglobulin to respond to antigenic stimulus, is well suited because of its structure as a bacterial agglutinator and complement mediator. IgA is seen mostly in seromucous secretions, where it serves as the major defender against bacteria. IgD most likely serves as an antigen receptor on lymphocyte surfaces, while IgE responds to parasitic infection and mediates allergic reactions, such as atopic allergy.

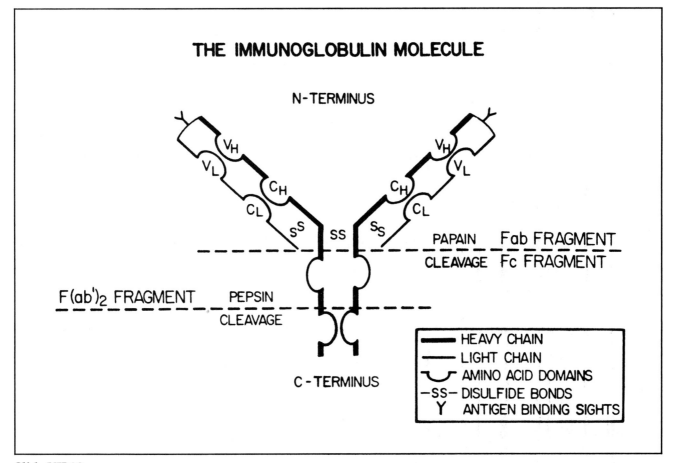

THE IMMUNOGLOBULIN MOLECULE

N-TERMINUS

PAPAIN Fab FRAGMENT
CLEAVAGE Fc FRAGMENT

F(ab')2 FRAGMENT   PEPSIN
CLEAVAGE

C - TERMINUS

— HEAVY CHAIN
— LIGHT CHAIN
⌣ AMINO ACID DOMAINS
-SS- DISULFIDE BONDS
Y ANTIGEN BINDING SIGHTS

Slide VII,28

The Immune Response

The humoral and cellular responses to antigen are closely related. Recent studies have identified two subpopulations of T cells. The suppressor cell appears to inhibit antibody production by B cells, while the helper cell enhances humoral responses. For any immune reaction to occur, however, antigen must first be processed, which takes place when macrophages phagocytose the antigens. The information derived from the foreign protein is then relayed to the B and T cells. This information is in the form of antigen cleaved to immunogenic fragments. These molecules may interact with RNA to form substances capable of carrying immunologic information to lymphocytes, or they may be transmitted to B or T cells as modified antigens.

As outlined in Slide VII,29, the humoral response to antigens (B-cell response) involves the synthesis and secretion of antibody to neutralize bacterial toxins and bacteria to expedite their removal. The T-cell response, or cell-mediated immune reaction, depends on the production of specific, sensitized lymphocytes with immunoglobulins on their surface. These lymphocytes secrete small effector molecules called lymphokines that are responsible for transplantation immunity and delayed hypersensitivity. Slide VII,30 summarizes the cell-mediated response to specific antigens.

The small lymphocyte is necessary to both cellular and humoral reactions. Without this cell, a primary antibody response to antigens such as tetanus toxoid cannot be mounted. These lymphocytes also carry the "memory" of the first coded contact with antigen.

In the humoral response, nonsensitized cells respond to antigens by a process called blastogenesis. The cells undergo a morphologic and metabolic transformation, with participation of the T helper cell. The B cell is transformed into a B lymphoblast. This phase of the immune response is called the afferent phase (Slide VII,30). The B lymphoblast may then become a plasma cell that produces a specific immunoglobulin. In addition, the B blast cell may become a memory cell in the phase known as the efferent arc (Slide VII,30). In the humoral response, specific antibody is the effector molecule that neutralizes the antigen.

In the cellular response, the T cell is the primary cell that responds to the antigen and acts as the effector arm. Specific antigens stimulate T-cell blastogenesis. They may become effector cells or memory cells. The cell-mediated response is summarized in Slide VII,30. Macrophages are involved in both the afferent response (production of T blast cells and the efferent response (production of cytotoxic T cells, memory cells, helper cells, suppressor cells). The cytotoxic cells (K cells) secrete lymphokines that may inhibit macrophages and influence lymphocytes or other targets such as viruses. The entire response system is directed by genetic codes that determine cell-surface antigens, response to antigens, and the alloantigenic differences between serum immunoglobulins.

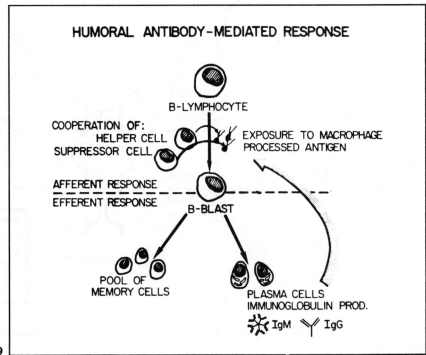

Slide VII,29

Tolerance and Autoimmunity

It is now recognized that immune pathways play a major role in the pathophysiology of many connective tissue diseases. This role is elucidated by the concepts of tolerance and autoimmunity.

Tolerance is immunologic unresponsiveness to autoantigens, which is a naturally occurring phenomenon that develops during fetal life. It is a recognition of "self" by immunocompetent lymphocytes induced by the exposure of lymphocytes to antigens. During adulthood, tolerance can develop following the administration of high doses of antigen. Tolerance is maintained by both the T and B cells and interactions of suppressor and helper T cells.

The breakdown of tolerance produces autoimmunity. While the exact mechanism responsible for the loss of self-recognition is not yet understood, several explanations have been proposed. One explanation proposes that sequestered antigens not encountered during fetal life are exposed; lymphocytes would respond to the previously sequestered antigens as they would to a foreign protein. Exposure of so-called immunologically privileged structures, such as chondrocytes and nucleoproteins, antigenic determinants hidden within proteins, may result from adjunctive disease processes.

Another mechanism of autoimmunity may be the alteration of previously tolerated antigens by viruses or other exogenous materials. As a result, lymphocytes no longer recognize the protein as "self." Similar to this mechanism is cross-reactivity, which occurs when a foreign antigen is structurally quite similar to a native antigen; antibodies produced in response to the foreign antigen cross-react to destroy the native, previously tolerated antigen. Another explanation for autoimmunity is that a normal lymphocyte undergoes mutation, producing mutant cells incapable of normal surveillance; instead, these cells interact with normal protein to produce autoantibodies. A final explanation involves defects arising in subpopulations of T cells. The suppressor cells become defective and are no longer able to restrain the helper cells, which results in the unchecked stimulation of antibodies, including autoantibodies.

Regardless of the mechanism responsible for the loss of tolerance, the result is the production of immune destructive mechanisms directed against "self." The orthopaedist is encountering immunologic disorders with increasing frequency.

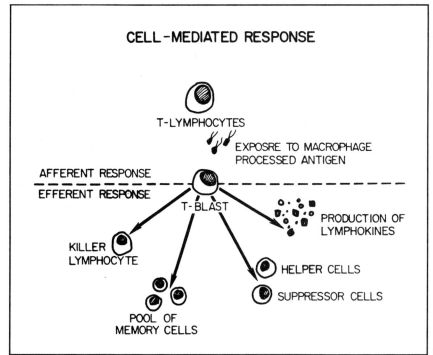

Slide VII,30

Selected Bibliography

Thromboembolic Disease

Asher M (ed): Orthopaedic Knowledge Update I. Chicago, American Academy of Orthopaedic Surgeons, 1984.

Bergquist D: Dextran and homeostasis, a review. Acta Chir Scand 1982; 148: 633-640.

Cranley JJ, Canos AJ, Sull WJ: The diagnosis of deep venous thrombosis. Fallibility of clinical symptoms and signs. Arch Surg 1976; 3: 34-36.

DeLee J, Rockwood CA, Jr: Current Concepts Review, the use of aspirin in thromboembolic disease. J Bone Joint Surg 1980; 62-A: 149-152.

Evarts CM: Thromboembolic Disease. Instructional Course Lectures. St. Louis, CV Mosby, 1979, vol 28, pp 67-71.

Gallus AS, Hirsh J: Treatment of venous thromboembolic disease. Seminars in thrombosis and hemostasis 1976; 2:291-331.

Greenfield LJ: Pulmonary embolism: Diagnosis and management. Current Prob in Surg 1976; 12:1-52.

Gruber UF, et al: Incidences of fatal postoperative pulmonary embolism after prophylaxis with dextran 70 and low-dose heparin; an international multicentre study. Br Med J 1980; 2:69-72.

Harris WH, et al: Aspirin prophylaxis of venous thromboembolism. New England J Med 1977; 297: 1246-1248.

Harris WH, Salzman EW, DeSanctis RW, et al: Prevention of venous thromboembolism following total hip replacement. 1972; JAMA 220:1319-1322.

Kakkar V. The diagnosis of deep vein thrombosis using the 125-I fibrinogen test. Arch Surg 1972; 104: 152-159.

Smith JB: The prostanoids in hemostasis and thrombosis: A review. Am J Path 1980; 99:743-804.

Stamatakis JD, et al: Failure of aspirin to prevent postoperative deep vein thrombosis in patients undergoing total hip replacement. Br Med J 1978; 1:1031-1032.

Wintrobe MM (ed): Clinical Hematology. Philadelphia, Lea and Febiger, 1981.

Shock

Goldfarb RD: Evaluation of ventricular performance in shock. Circ Shock 1985; 15(4):281-301.

Lane PL, McLellan BA, Johns PD: Etiology of shock in blunt trauma. Can Med Assoc J 1985; 133(3):199-201.

MacLean LD: Shock: Causes and management of circulatory collapse, in Sabiston DC, Jr (ed): Davis-Christopher Textbook of Surgery, ed 12. Philadelphia, WB Saunders, 1981, pp 58-90.

Adult Respiratory Distress Syndrome

Amato JJ, Rhinelander HF, Cleveland RJ: Post-traumatic adult respiratory distress syndrome. Orth Clin N Amer 1978; 9:693-713.

Gossling HR, Pellegrini VD, Jr: Fat embolism syndrome: a review of the pathophysiology and physiological basis of treatment. Clin Orthop 1982; 165: 68-82.

Montgomery AB, Stager MA, Carrico CJ, et al: Causes of mortality in patients with Adult Respiratory Distress Syndrome. Am Rev Respir Dis 1985; 132: 485-489.

Moore FD, et al: Post-Traumatic Pulmonary Insufficiency. Philadelphia, WB Saunders, 1969.

Riede U, Sandritter W, Mittermeyer C: Circulatory shock: A review. Pathology 1981; 13(2):299-311.

Riseborough EJ, Herndon JH, Alterations in pulmonary function, coagulation and fat metabolism in patients with fractures of the lower limbs. Clin Orthop 1976; 2:248-267.

Shapiro BA, Cane RD, Harrison RA: Positive end-expiratory pressure therapy in adults with special reference to acute lung injury: A review of the literature and suggested clinical corrections. Crit Care Med 1984; 12(2):27-41.

Shapiro BA, Harrison RA, Trout CA: Clinical Application of Respiratory Care, ed 2. Chicago, Year Book Medical Publishers Inc, 1979, pp 93-97.

Hemoglobinopathies

Bunn HF, Forget BG, Ranney HM: Hemoglobinopathies, in Smith LH(ed): Major Problems in Internal Medicine. Philadelphia, WB Saunders, 1977, vol 12.

Diggs LW: Bone and joint lesions in sickle cell disease. Clin Orthop 1967; 52:119.

Huisman THJ: Normal and abnormal hemgloblin. Adv Clin Chem 1972; 15:149.

Wintrobe MM (ed): Clinical Hematology. Philadelphia, Lea and Febiger, 1981.

Pathophysiology of Musculoskeletal Sepsis

Asher MM (ed): Orthopaedic Knowledge Update I. Chicago, American Academy of Orthopaedic Surgeons, 1984.

Roca RP, Yoshikawa TT: Primary skeletal infections in heroin users: a clinical characterization, diagnosis and therapy. Clin Orthop 1979; 144:238-248.

Immunobiology

The section on Immunobiology in Chapter 7 has been used with permission of Victor M. Goldberg, M.D. and the W. B. Saunders Company, publisher of *Osteoarthritis Diagnosis and Management*. See listing below.

Goldberg VM: The immunology of articular cartilage, in Moskowitz, Goldberg, Mankin: Osteoarthritis Diagnosis and Management. Philadelphia, WB Saunders, 1984, pp 81-85.

Illustration and Slide Index

The illustration and slide index gives a brief description of each slide in the set and corresponding illustration found in the syllabus. The index is organized by chapter, with each entry listed in numerical order.

Where appropriate, the entry lists not only the content of the slide, but the type of slide, e.g., photomicrograph or radiograph. Because the slides for Biomechanics, Biomaterials, and Non-skeletal Disorders consist almost entirely of tables, graphs, or diagrams, the slide type has been omitted for these entries.

Anatomy

1. Diagrams—types of bone
2. Photomicrograph—woven and lamellar bone
3. Photomicrograph—bone osteon
4. Photomicrograph—cortical bone
5. Electron photomicrograph—vessels in haversian canal
6. Photomicrograph— vasculature of cortical bone
7. Light and electron photomicrographs—osteoblasts
8. Electron photomicrograph—mature osteocyte
9. Light and electron photomicrograph—osteoclasts
10. Illustration—Hydroxyapatite
11. Electron photomicrograph—bone collagen
12. Diagram—scheme for initial calcification
13. Diagram—mineral accretion
14. Diagram—enchondral bone development
15. Diagram—growth plate (physis)
16. Diagram—blood supply of the growth plate
17. Diagram—zones of the cartilaginous portion of the growth plate
18. Composite electron photomicrographs—calcium-stained mitochondria in growth plate
19. Diagram—metabolic events in the growth plate
20. Photomicrograph—growth plate (P.A.S./Alcian blue stain)
21. Diagram—proteoglycan aggregates in growth plate
22. Electron photomicrograph—matrix vesicles
23. Diagram—summary of cartilage mineralization
24. Composite photomicrograph and diagram—metaphysis
25. Photomicrograph and diagram—ossification groove of Ranvier and perichondrial ring of LaCroix
26. Histologic and radiographic features—achondroplasia
27. Histologic and radiographic features—rickets
28. Diagram—vascular loops in rickets
29. Histologic and radiographic features—Osteogenesis imperfecta
30. Histologic and radiographic features—osteopetrosis
31. Composite—adult articular cartilage
32. Diagram and photomicrograph—articular cartilage
33. Diagram—compressed and expanded proteoglycan aggregate.
34. Diagram—proteoglycan aggregate
35. Diagram—proteoglycan molecule and its subunits in collagen matrix
36. Electron photomicrograph—collagen fibril network and proteoglycan aggregates
37. Diagram—"swelling pressure" in articular cartilage
38. Photomicrograph and schematic representation—Hultkrantz split line pattern in distal femoral condyle
39. Diagram—collagen fibers in the menisci
40. Electron photomicrograph—collagen bundles
41. Scanning electron photomicrograph—collagen bundles
42. Photomicrograph—blood supply to the knee meniscus
43. Diagram—muscle fiber orientation
44. Diagram—breakdown of a muscle from gross muscle level to myofilament level
45. Photomicrograph—skeletal muscle
46. Composite—connective tissue components of skeletal muscle
47. Histochemical preparation—skeletal muscle
48. Table—properties of fiber types
49. Table—enzymatic properties of fiber types
50. Table—physical properties of fiber types
51. Electron photomicrograph—ultrastructure of myofibrils
52. Table—characteristics of nerve fibers
53. Diagram—innervation of skeletal muscle
54. Photomicrograph—motor unit
55. Electron photomicrograph—motor end plate
56. Electron photomicrograph—satellite cell of skeletal muscle
57. Diagram—Blix length-tension curve
58. Photomicrograph—tendon-bone interface
59. Photomicrograph—tendon
60. Electron photomicrograph—tendon collagen

61. Diagram—tendon structure
62. Diagram—Healing tendon within sheath
63. Photograph—vincula of tendon
64. Photomicrograph—intrinsic blood supply of tendon
65. Photomicrograph—cross section of peripheral nerve
66. Electron photomicrograph—peripheral nerve myelin sheath
67. Electron photomicrograph—nodes of Ranvier

Disorders of Bone

1. Composite—lines of force on head and neck of femur
2. Composite—effects of age on metacarpal cortex and femoral diaphysis
3. Schematic drawing—principles of bone remodeling
4. Microradiograph—dynamics of bone remodeling
5. Photomicrograph—cutting cones' mechanism
6. Diagram—metabolic pathways of vitamin D
7. Diagram—calcium homeostasis
8. Graph—calcium requirements by age
9. Graph—relationship among bone mass, age and sex
10. Composite—osteopenic states; bone biopsy technique
11. Photomicrograph—hyperparathyroidism
12. Diagram—pathogenesis of bone changes in renal osteodystrophy
13. Composite radiographs—osteomalacia
14. Radiograph—renal osteodystrophy
15. Graph—bone mass regulation by hormones
16. Photomicrograph—changes in cortical thickness of bone with osteoporosis
17. Diagram—calcium metabolism in osteoporosis
18. Diagram—recommended treatments for osteoporosis
19. Composite—Paget's disease
20. Photomicrograph—pagetoid vertebral body
21. Photomicrograph—bone repair: inflammatory stage
22. Photomicrograph—bone repair: soft callus stage, increased vascularity
23. Photomicrograph—bone repair: soft callus stage, new cartilage formation
24. Photomicrograph—bone repair: hard callus stage
25. Photomicrograph—primary bone healing
26. Photomicrograph—blood flow at fracture site
27. Diagram—changes in oxygen tension at fracture site
28. Composite photomicrograph—nonunion vs. early-healing callus
29. Composite photomicrograph—transition from cancellous bone graft to reconstituted bone
30. Composite photomicrograph—creeping substitution (top)—necrotic bone (left) —new bone formation (right)—cross-section of fibular graft (bottom)
31. Pedigree chart—autosomal dominant inheritance pattern
32. Pedigree chart—autosomal recessive inheritance pattern
33. Pedigree chart—sex-linked dominant inheritance pattern
34. Pedigree chart—sex-linked recessive inheritance pattern
35. Composite diagram—polygenic inheritance

Soft-Tissue Disorders

1. Diagram—composition of connective tissue
2. Diagram—composition of collagen fibrils
3. Table—composition of fibrillar collagens
4. Diagram—composition of proteoglycan
5. Diagram—glycosaminoglycans
6. Diagram—proteoglycans with and without compression
7. Photomicrograph—structure of proteoglycan aggregates
8. Electron photomicrograph—proteoglycan aggregates
9. Table—the glycoproteins in hyaline cartilage
10. Diagram—assemblage of proteoglycan aggregates
11. Graph—water content by depth of articular cartilage
12. Graph—collagen content by depth of articular cartilage
13. Photomicrograph—lacerated articular cartilage, not full thickness
14. Photomicrograph—full thickness injury of articular cartilage
15. Photomicrograph—repair matrix of articular cartilage
16. Photomicrograph—degeneration of repair cartilage
17. Photomicrograph—immobilized joint: cartilage thinning
18. Photomicrograph—immobilized joint: fibrofatty tissue

Pathology

35. Radiograph—osteochondral exostosis
36. Gross specimen—osteochondral exostosis
37. Table—staging
38. Table—surgical margins and staging
39. Computed axial tomography—lipoma in axilla
40. Photomicrograph—pseudocapsule
41. Diagram—tumor invading muscle
42. Gross specimen—soft tissue sarcoma
43. Gross specimen—soft tissue sarcoma invading muscle
44. Photomicrograph—sarcoma dissecting between muscle fibers
45. Schematic representation—abscess development: Epiphyseal plate
46. Radiograph—osteomyelitis
47. Photomicrograph—osteomyelitis
48. Radiographs—osteomyelitis
49. Hemisection—normal femur of a child
50. Radiograph—osteomyelitis in child's hip
51. Gross specimen—osteomyelitis: Involucrum in femur
52. Radiograph—osteomyelitis in fibula: Sequestrum surrounded by involucrum
53. Photomicrograph—osteomyelitis
54. Photomicrograph—involucrum
55. Photomicrograph—rheumatoid arthritis
56. Gross specimen—rheumatoid tenosynovitis
57. Radiograph—rheumatoid arthritis
58. Photomicrograph—rheumatoid synovium
59. Photomicrograph—rheumatoid nodule
60. Radiograph—podagra
61. Photomicrograph—gout
62. Photomicrograph—gouty synovitis
63. Photomicrograph (polarized light)—urate crystal
64. Photomicrograph—tuberculous granuloma
65. Radiograph—chondrocalcinosis
66. Photomicrograph—calcium pyrophosphate crystal
67. Radiograph—pigmented villonodular synovitis
68. Gross specimen—pigmented villonodular synovitis
69. Radiograph—synovial osteochondromatosis
70. Gross specimen—synovial osteochondromatosis
71. Photomicrograph—synovial osteochondromatosis
72. Radiograph—hemophilic arthropathy
73. Gross specimen—hemophilic arthropathy

74. Photomicrograph—osteonecrosis
75. Photomicrograph—osteonecrosis
76. Photomicrograph—osteonecrosis
77. Radiograph—osteonecrosis
78. Diagram—osteonecrosis seen in previous radiograph
79. Gross specimen—osteonecrotic femur
80. Photograph of coronal sections—osteonecrosis
81. Gross specimen—osteochondritis dissecans
82. Photomicrograph—osteonecrosis (cutting cone)
83. Photomicrograph—osteonecrosis: Later stage (cutting cone)

Biomechanics

1. Definition of force
2. Definition of moment
3. Static equilibrium
4. Forces at the hip joint: Free body diagram
5. Forces on the hip
6. Forces on the spine
7. Forces on the shoulder
8. Forces on the knee
9. Forces on the ankle
10. Translations and rotations
11. Contact surface motion
12. Definition of stress
13. Definition of strain
14. Material versus structural behavior
15. Cortical bone: Directional properties
16. Cortical bone: Fatigue failure
17. Trabecular bone: Effects of apparent density
18. Cortical bone: Effects of aging
19. Ligaments and tendons: Material properties
20. Material properties of various soft tissues
21. Bone-ligament complex: Structural properties
22. Ligament trauma: Effects of strain rates
23. Meniscus: Directional properties
24. Intervertebral disc: Viscoelastic creep
25. Intervertebral disc: Viscoelastic stress relaxation
26. Cartilage and meniscus: Flow-dependent creep
27. Ligaments: Material versus structural properties
28. Ligaments: Material versus structural properties
29. Femur: Bending

Non-skeletal Disorders

1. Incidence of death for pulmonary embolism
2. Frequency of deep-vein thrombosis
3. Blood coagulation mechanism
4. Fibrinolytic mechanisms
5. Platelet nidus formation
6. Role of factor X in thrombin formation
7. Pathogenesis of postoperative venous thrombosis
8. Diagnostic methods: Venous thrombosis
9. Diagnostic steps: Venous thrombosis
10. Blood coagulation mechanism: Effect of coumadin
11. Pharmaceutical agents: Thrombus dissolution
12. Compensatory reactions in shock
13. Compensatory reactions in shock
14. Blood volume restitution in shock
15. Changes in renal function following trauma
16. Fluid shifts in hemorrhagic shock
17. Effect of fluid replacement on survival in hemorrhagic shock
18. Potassium shifts in hemorrhagic shock
19. Ventilation/perfusion abnormalities
20. Possible causes of ARDS following injury
21. Photomicrograph—fat globules in the lung
22. Pathologic events in the fat embolism syndrome
23. Electron photomicrograph—lung surfactant
24. Distribution of hemoglobin genotypes
25. Pathogenesis of bone infarct in sickle-cell disease
26. Characteristics of the immune system
27. Origins of immunocompetent cells
28. Structural units of the immunoglobulin molecule
29. Humoral antibody-mediated response
30. Cell-mediated response

Index